PSYCHIATRY
AND
GENERAL PRACTICE

*Based on the proceedings of a Conference
held in Oxford 11 – 13 September, 1981
Published for the Mental Health Foundation*

PSYCHIATRY
AND
GENERAL PRACTICE

Edited by

ANTHONY W. CLARE
MALCOLM LADER

Institute of Psychiatry
Denmark Hill, London

1982

ACADEMIC PRESS

A Subsidiary of Harcourt Brace Jovanovich, Publishers

London   New York

Paris   San Diego   San Francisco   São Paulo

Sydney   Tokyo   Toronto

ACADEMIC PRESS INC. (LONDON) LTD.
24/28 Oval Road
London NW1

United States Edition published by
ACADEMIC PRESS INC.
111 Fifth Avenue
New York, New York 10003

British Library Cataloguing in Publication Data
Psychiatry and General Practice.
1. Psychiatry—Congresses
I. Clare, A. W.   II. Lader, M.
616.89   RC454

ISBN 0-12-174720-4

Printed by St Edmundsbury Press, Bury St Edmunds, Suffolk

CONTRIBUTORS

ASHTON, John R. *Department of Community Health, London School of Hygiene and Tropical Medicine, Keppel Street (Gower Street), London WC1E 7HT.*

ASHURST, Pamela M. *Department of Psychotherapy, Royal South Hants Hospital, Graham Road, Southampton SO9 4PE.*

CLARE, Anthony W. *Institute of Psychiatry, De Crespigny Park, Denmark Hill, London SE5 8AF.*

COOPER, John E. *Professorial Unit, Mapperley Hospital, Porchester Road, Nottingham NG3 6AA.*

CORNEY, Roslyn H. *Institute of Psychiatry, De Crespigny Park, Denmark Hill, London SE5 8AF.*

FRY, John *138 Croydon Road, Beckenham, Kent BR3 4DG.*

GOLDBERG, David *Department of Psychiatry, The University Hospital of South Manchester, West Didsbury, Manchester M20 8LR.*

HORDER, John *The Royal College of General Practitioners, 14 Prince's Gate, London SW7 1PU.*

INGHAM, Jack *MRC Unit for Epidemiological Studies in Psychiatry, University Department of Psychiatry, Royal Edinburgh Hospital, Morningside Park, Edinburgh EH10 5HF.*

PARISH, Peter A. *Medicines Research Unit, 32 Park Place, Cardiff CF1 3BA.*

SABBAGH, Karl *MSD Foundation, Tavistock Square, London WC1H 9LG.*

SHEPHERD, Michael *Department of Epidemiology, The Institute of Psychiatry, De Crespigny Park, Denmark Hill, London SE5 8AF.*

ZANDER, Luke *General Practice Teaching and Research Unit, St. Thomas' Hospital Medical School, 80 Kennington Road, London SE11 4TH.*

THE MENTAL HEALTH FOUNDATION

The Mental Health Foundation is Britain's leading grant-making charity concerned with promoting, encouraging and financing pioneering research and community care projects.

It aims to prevent mental disorders by awarding Fellowships and Grants for research into the causes and treatment of mental illness and handicap; improving the quality of life for the mentally disordered by supporting pioneering and innovative care schemes; rehabilitating those who have suffered from mental illness by encouraging new projects in the fields of employment, housing and self-help in the community.

FOREWORD

*(Based on a speech given at the Conference Dinner by
Sir George Young, the then Parliamentary Under Secretary of
State for Health).*

The subject chosen for your Conference is a crucial one,
Psychiatry and General Practice, and it links very closely
with three major policy priorities that the Department is
pursuing.

We are committed to giving greater priority to the Cinder-
ella services, of which mental health is a major item. For
various reasons mental health has not been receiving its
rightful share of the resources, and we are determined to put
that right. I welcome the work of the London Health Planning
Consortium which has shown how acute hospital services in
London have in fact developed preferentially while psychiatric
services and primary health have lagged behind. One of the
ways to give mental health greater priority is not to regard
it as a service apart, but to ensure that it is an integral
part of health and social service provision.

The second reason why this coincides with our policy
priority is our emphasis on prevention. Like the development
of the mental health service, we set this out in some detail
in "Care in Action" published earlier this year. Again the
links between prevention, mental health and general practice
are apparent.

Our third policy area is our commitment to community care.
Recently one of my main concerns has been the difficulties
which the inevitable distinction between the NHS on the one
hand and personal social services on the other have presented
in many areas, but particularly mental health. So we published
a Green Paper in July 1981, "Care in the Community", which
identifies ways of surmounting these difficulties. That
document discussed a whole range of means of switching
resources from the NHS to community care, where that is
appropriate and right for the patient.

So that general background explains why the Government is
very interested in the theme of your Conference, and we hope
to push forward as fast as we can, placing greater emphasis

on primary care in mental health on co-operation between the
primary care teams and specialists of the voluntary organizations: that co-operation is absolutely crucial. It has been
appreciated that primary care is the biggest provider in terms
of services for the mentally ill, but the recent book by
Goldberg and Huxley (1981) has made that more apparent. It
also discusses the pathway to better psychiatric care, and I
found very interesting their demonstration of the filter system which really brings home the dependence on GPs, and demon-
strates the very small proportion of cases that are treated by
a psychiatrist. At the same time, general practice itself is
changing, and the primary health care team is becoming much
stronger.

The Royal Commission commented on the importance of the
health visitor and one of the studies of Professor Shepherd
(Harwin, 1975) has shown how the skills of the district nurse
have really helped in identifying depression and problems
amongst the elderly.

So a great deal of progress has been made in improving
mental health provision but, of course, the climate is now
right for even greater progress and I very much welcome some
of the initiatives of the Royal College of General Practitioners, particularly the whole series of reports on prevention in general practice. I read a particularly excellent
one on the prevention of psychiatric disorders (RCGP, 1981),
and this report was one of the reasons for the Conference.
We are indebted to John Horder and the RCGP for their initiative and foresight in commissioning that particular report.

Of course, the specialist services have been moving into
community care for a very long time. About 80,000 patients
are now visited regularly by the hospital-based community
psychiatric nurses, and with the others who are attending the
day hospitals, the number currently receiving some form of
care from the specialist service is at least as high as it was
20 years ago. But from the point of view of primary care the
difference is that half of those people are now back at home
under the care of their GP. Of course, the doctors are no
longer fixed in their separate spheres. We had about 80,000
domiciliary visits by consultant psychiatrists in 1979, and
people have stressed to me both the importance of these visits
as learning experiences and that the learning is two-way. What
the psychiatrist learns from the GP is as important as what
the GP learns from the psychiatrist.

All this flexibility is excellent, but it raises many
questions about the nature of the relationship and the communication between the primary and specialist care. What of the
health centre, the day hospital and the day centre? Should

these be the points of close integration of the primary and
specialist care, and what is the role of social services in
all this?

But you ask, "What basically is the Government going to do
to help?" We make no claim to take over problems and solve
them automatically, but I can identify four aspects where the
Government's role may be helpful. One of these I have already
touched on, the Green Paper, "Care in the Community", which I
hope will pave the way for real advances towards community
care. Secondly, there is the Mental Health Act. We want to
introduce amending legislation during the life of the present
Parliament. The Act has served the country well and many
trends are already moving in the right direction. For example,
in the last 10 years the number of emergency admissions under
Section 29 has halved from 16,000 in 1970 to 8,000 in 1979.
But when we have amending legislation, we hope it can be
accompanied by changes to take into account the points that
have been made in the review of the Act about the training of
social workers approved for mental health work, and about a
code of practice for compulsory admissions, and both of these
should make for the smoother working of Part IV.

Then, of course, research, a key area where the Mental
Health Foundation and the Department have a very strong common
interest. We have given longstanding support to the General
Practice Research Unit of the Institute of Psychiatry, directed
by Professor Shepherd, and our full extent and the range of
our commitment to research in that field is set out in our
annual handbook of research and development (DHSS, 1981).

Finally, there is a need for training and education, a
complex area where the position differs across the disciplines.
So far as doctors are concerned, the main responsibility for
the content of training and education of doctors working in
mental health lies rightly with their professional bodies and
the universities. My Department's role is, with the advice
of the profession, to ensure that there are sufficient medical
training posts for the needs of the service, not just for the
consultants in psychiatry but also for doctors wishing to gain
experience in psychiatry before they go into general practice.
On top of that, we are providing money under Section 63 of
the Health Services and Public Health Act for the continuing
education of general practitioners, and that, of course, is
a key element in the transmission of the new practices in
psychiatric care which I have been talking about, and we are
putting about £1.5 million a year into that.

Can I acknowledge a still wider responsibility which rests
on Government and also on many others? Some activities, some
social structures, and some family patterns, seem to be helpful to mental health, in other words they reduce the likelihood

of problems, and reverse ones are harmful. Few findings in
this area are clearcut, but, for example, the argument about
high rise flats shows how badly we need some first class
research to investigate these very complex inter-relationships.
We need to involve the whole of society with concerns about
unemployment, about housing, about the environment, about
education and so on, and also to make institutions that now
exist - the Government included - far more sensitive to mental
health issues.

REFERENCES

DHSS (1981). "Handbook of Research and Development". HMSO.
Goldberg, D. and Huxley, P. (1981). "Mental Illness in the
     Community. The Pathway to Psychiatric Care". Tavistock,
     London.
Harwin, B. (1975). Psychiatric screening. *In* "Screening in
     General Practice" (Ed. C.R. Hart). Churchill Livingstone,
     London.
RCGP (1981). Prevention of psychiatric disorders in general
     practice. Report of a sub-Committee of the Royal College
     of General Practitioners' Working Party on Prevention.

PREFACE

In September 1979 the Mental Health Foundation held a conference devoted to the issue of psychiatric research, the speakers
being amongst the most distinguished research workers in the
country. A great many issues were discussed, from viral
immunology to psychotherapy, and the entire proceedings were
subsequently published (Lader, 1980). However, as more than
one perceptive critic observed, there was little mention of
the role of primary care, not merely in the management of
psychiatric ill-health, but in the task of elucidating its
nature, course and response to treatment. The conference
held in September 1981 not merely puts this omission to right,
but it complements neatly the earlier conference and helps
provide a rounded perspective of the state of psychological
medicine at the beginning of the 1980s.

Gathered together at Oxford in September 1981 were representatives not only of psychiatry and general practice but
also of the allied disciplines of social work, health visiting,
community medicine, nursing, psychology and of the relevant
divisions within the Department of Health and Social Security.
In the light of this diversity of background, it seems
reasonable to suggest that the opportunity provided by the
conference to review and assess two decades of research
relating to the identification and management of psychosocial
disorders in primary care and to highlight the potential for
future fruitful research was a unique one.

While the tripartite division of the conference proceedings
- epidemiology, treatment and organization of services -
served a useful function in ensuring that the contributions
and discussion were clearly focused throughout, the opening
paper by Dr Ingham quickly illustrates its arbitrariness.
One issue, touched on by him, namely the vexed question of
so-called "trivial complaints", reverberates throughout the
subsequent proceedings. Professor Parish speaks for many
when he warns against the medicalization of problems which
might be better conceptualized as "social" and "treated" by
non-medical means. However, even here, the absence of reli-
able data concerning the precise nature of such complaints,
not to mention their natural history and outcome whether

treated or not, only emphasizes Dr Clare's argument on behalf
of a system of problem recording more appropriate to the GP's
everyday requirements than current systems derived largely
from hospital practice. In the absence of data opinions bloom
only to wither away when data become available. Dr Fry's
contribution provides a timely example when he argues, on the
basis of data carefully accumulated over 20 and more years,
against the conventional wisdom which holds that psychological
distress and the consumption of psychotropic drugs have
increased dramatically in recent years. Fry's presentation
also serves to exemplify Professor Shepherd's delineation of
the potential research role of the general practitioner, a
role which can be carried out quite effectively with little
more than an age-sex register and records which lend themselves
to psychiatric analysis.

Nor need such research be unrelated to the day-to-day
realities of general practice. The contributions at this
conference relating to the management of psychiatric ill-
health in primary care illustrate both the needs and the
possibilities. Dr Zander unashamedly proclaims the value of
the GP working within a multi-disciplinary primary care team
but he is at pains to couple this popular message with a less
commonly voiced plea on behalf of a more economic use of such
resources so that each team member functions to the very
optimum of his or her potential. The two research contributions on the role of social workers and counsellors illustrate
his point perfectly. Dr Corney's meticulously designed and
carefully mounted study indicates what can and cannot be
expected from social work intervention in the management of
acute depression. Dr Ashurst's paper, too, implicitly endorses
the need more carefully to match patient and treatment.
While she is, perhaps, understandably enthusiastic about the
value of counselling, problems of design, patient selection,
matching and outcome measures in her study together with what
must be seen as a disappointing lack of counselling impact on
surgery attendances, psychotropic drug prescribing and overall
response caution against excessive zeal and expectations in
this area.

The attachment of different professionals, however, only
adds further impetus to the pressing need to clarify the role,
actual and potential, of the psychiatrist. We still know
pitifully little about the factors which influence GP referral
patterns and one possible fruit of the kinds of collaborative
venture proposed by Professor Cooper is clarification of where
the boundary between what is the proper preserve of the
specialised psychiatric service and that of general practice
might best be drawn. Once again, the research possibilities
raised by differing methods of general practice-psychiatry

collaboration are numerous. What will be the impact on
referral patterns and referral rates of such collaborative
arrangements? What, if any, will be the effects on psychotropic drug prescribing, GP attitudes towards psychiatric
disorders, GP tolerance of so-called "trivial complaints"?
Will closer collaboration improve the GP's diagnostic sensi-
tivities and skills, so neatly dissected and analysed by
Professor Goldberg? And with Dr Ashton's contribution we
return once again to the inter-relationship between social
factors and policy on the one hand and the ideology and practice of medicine on the other, leaving us with the question:
Is it our intention to improve primary care and deploy its
resources so as to make the diagnosis and management of the
physical, psychological and social distress that present
there as good as it can possibly be or do we want to train
our doctors so that they can screen out those "social" problems
which some of the Oxford participants believe have no business
appearing in the general practice surgery?

And whichever kind of GP we want, who should do the training? And what should be taught? And where? The video consultation exercise undertaken by Anthony Clare and Karl
Sabbagh at this conference demonstrated the very different
perspectives on the doctor-patient relationship held by the
GP and the psychiatrist. The psychiatrist, accustomed to
obtaining much of his information from his patient in the
course of one or at most two lengthy interviews is often
shocked by the apparent cursoriness of the general practice
consultation. The GP, familiar with building up a picture
not merely of his patient but of the patient's personal,
social and occupational circumstances on the basis of a number
of short but related contacts, is exasperated by the psychiatrist's somewhat cavalier attitude to that scarce commodity,
time. The responses of the conference participants to the
video highlighted these differences and, in addition, served
to warn against a too hasty assumption that we know all we
need to know about what is a "good" interview, what are
"appropriate" interventions, what is the "correct" pose to be
adopted by the general practitioner and what it is that leads
to a reasonably satisfactory outcome.

Professor Shepherd, winding up the conference, strikes an
apt note. "The case for intensive investigation along a broad
front has now been established" he remarks apropos the possibilities and challenges in the area of general practice
psychiatry, "but it must be acknowledged that so far we have
barely scratched the surface". It is the fervent hope of the
Mental Health Foundation, a hope which led to the holding of
this conference, that the energy and interest so evident in

Oxford can be so channelled as to produce over the next two
decades some much more substantial excavations.

REFERENCE

Lader, M. (1980). "Priorities in Psychiatric Research".
    John Wiley, Chichester.

Anthony W. Clare and Malcolm Lader
March, 1982.

CONTENTS

SESSION II

SESSION III

SESSION I

EPIDEMIOLOGY OF PSYCHIATRIC ILLNESS IN GENERAL PRACTICE

Opening Address given by Dr John Horder,
President of the Royal College of General Practitioners.

The CHAIRMAN: I welcome you all to this beautiful city and this lovely College on this particularly fine morning. I particularly welcome two visitors, Dr Barbara Burns from the National Institute of Mental Health in Washington, and Dr June Huntington from Sydney, Australia. May I thank the Mental Health Foundation not only for organizing this Conference but also for their support of my own College in publishing the Report on the Prevention of Psychiatric Disorders in General Practice (1981).

First, who are we? Most are general practitioners, the next largest contingent being psychiatrists. But there are at least 11 different professional groups here. We should not think of ourselves only as professional groups but also as ordinary people, even potential patients. The broadest view of psychiatry spreads to the problems of almost all ordinary families. The narrow view of psychiatry regards it as such a difficult subject for general practitioners that they need the help of all the other groups here, not just psychiatrists.

Why this Conference? It reflects a realization that general practitioners do need help in this subject. The interest of GPs in the subject has increased over the last 25 years and it may be that their skill has also increased. There has certainly been more training. My personal prejudice is that in the past our profession underestimated the importance of mental pain as against physical pain. Central to the training of the general practitioner is the combination of general medicine and psychiatry.

I have three questions. First, are GPs really more interested in this subject than they used to be? If one believes Dr Ann Cartwright's recent report (Cartwright and Anderson, 1981) and an even more very recent report, then there is doubt about this.

The second concerns the preventive psychiatry report which my College recently produced (1981). Are we realistic in supposing that prevention in this area is possible? Do we know enough about the principles of mental health, for instance, to advise mothers in our baby clinics, or even to discuss the problems with them, let alone advise? Is it worthwhile to intervene early in depressive or anxiety states?

The last question is how much of this work should the GP himself undertake? To what extent should we share it with those who work with us; to what extent should we be moving towards self-help groups? Fortunately, it is only my job to ask questions and not to try to answer them. That is the task of the speakers.

REFERENCES

Cartwright, A. and Anderson, R. (1981). General Practice Revisited: A Second Study of Patients and their Doctors. Tavistock, London.
Prevention of Psychiatric Disorders in General Practice. (1981). Report of a sub-Committee of the Royal College of General Practitioners' Working Party on Prevention. RCGP.

DEFINING THE PROBLEM

Jack Ingham

*MRC Unit for Epidemiological Studies
in Psychiatry, University Department of Psychiatry,
Royal Edinburgh Hospital, Morningside Park,
Edinburgh EH10 5HF*

It is to be hoped that for most primary care health workers
it is no longer necessary to convince them of the importance
of psychological problems amongst their patients. The object
of this paper is to make 3 simple points. Some people may
consider them too simple, but I believe it is necessary to
make and repeat them as they are vitally important. The first
is that the majority of psychological problems seen in
primary care consulters are not illnesses. This may seem an
obvious point, but words like pathology, mental illness and
mental disorder are still very widely used in this context.
Secondly, it is bad for patients who suffer from psychological problems, but are not mentally sick, to believe they
are ill. Thirdly, there is as yet no satisfactory way of
distinguishing clearly between patients with normal psychological problems and those who really are sick, except in
extreme cases. There is a large grey borderline area of
patients in distress who may be ill or in the process of
becoming ill, but equally may be experiencing normal emotional
reactions in difficult circumstances, reactions that are
unpleasant but can be coped with.

Epidemiological studies have played their part in providing convincing evidence of the importance of psychological
problems in the GP's workload. Doctors are certainly more
aware of psychological disorders now than they were a generation ago. Now the important questions are about the nature
of the problems and how they should be dealt with. Family
doctors detect the problems well enough, but are often
bewildered in deciding what to do about them and they seek
in vain for clear practical advice. This tends to lead to
one of three extreme types of response. The first is pill-
pushing, prescribing tranquillizers or tricyclics to everyone

who has an emotional problem, the second is referring everyone to the psychiatrist in an attempt to pass the buck, and
the third is do-it-yourself psychotherapy. These are
obviously 3 caricatures rather than representing what any
real doctors do in practice, but the tendencies do exist in
various combinations and most doctors wonder if they are
doing the best thing for their patients. The people who might
be able to advise them, e.g. clinical psychologists and
psychiatrists, are hampered by the fact that they do not know
enough about the nature of the problem. They tend to think
in terms of psychiatric out-patients and in-patients but the
problems arising in primary care are different.

First, how big a problem is it? This is the question that
most epidemiological studies are directed towards. What is
the prevalence of psychiatric illness in the community, particularly amongst those who seek the help of their GPs?
Before we can find out, we need to know what psychiatric illness is and achieving a usable operational definition has
proved a troublesome problem. This has led in the past to
enormous variations between morbidity rates reported by different investigators. Shepherd and his colleagues reviewed
this area in 1966 (Shepherd *et al.*, 1966) and found 20
studies which gave morbidity rates varying from 3.7% at the
lower end to 65% at the top. This was an astounding variation, but some of it could be accounted for by different
sampling methods, different definitions of the population,
or different periods of time over which prevalence was
assessed. Even allowing for all of these things the discrepancies were still pretty enormous, but at that time there
was no standard psychiatric interview procedure or questionnaire that could be applied on a large scale in a general
population survey and also provide an acceptable criterion
for detecting psychiatric illness. Most of the studies used
unspecified clinical interviewing procedures carried out
either by the general practitioners themselves, or by collaborating psychiatric experts. Since then quite a number of
standardized and, to some extent, validated instruments have
been developed and results are now appearing.

In developing a case finding instrument suitable for use
in a population survey, there are 2 very substantial difficulties. First psychiatric diagnosis is based largely on
what patients say about their feelings. Many of the feelings
they describe can be experienced by anyone, including those
who are not sick, albeit less intensely or under more extreme
circumstances. To take one example, there is an arbitrary
element in deciding how intensely and under what circumstances
a feeling of sadness must be experienced to be considered

abnormal. Secondly, the interview on which psychiatric diagnosis is generally based in clinics and hospitals depends a
great deal upon the subjective judgement of the skilled and
experienced clinician using unstructured procedures. It is
obviously unrealistic to expect consistent results over different investigations unless there is some standardization of
procedure and several centres have attempted to achieve this.
Two main contenders in the past few years have been the
Medical Research Council Unit at the Institute of Psychiatry
under Professor Wing (Wing *et al.*, 1974) and on the other
side of the Atlantic, the Biometrics Research Division of New
York State in which Spitzer and colleagues have been involved
(Spitzer and Endicott, 1978). Wing's team has produced the
Present State Examination (PSE) which is an attempt to produce a standardized interview, as similar as possible to a
normal psychiatric clinical interview, with the questions and
coding instructions sufficiently specified to enable all
observers trained in the technique to arrive at the same
result. A lot of research effort has been invested in this
technique and there is now abundant evidence of its reliability
in the hands of trained and experienced clinicians. Its
American counterpart is called the Schedule for Affective
Disorders and Schizophrenia (SADS) and was devised with
similar aims. It also has reasonably satisfactory reliability.
One disadvantage of both methods as originally devised, is
that they could only be used by experienced clinicians. In
addition to the standard questions that are asked of every-
body, skillful probing is required before a symptom can be
coded as definitely present and this part of the procedure
requires a lot of clinical skill and judgement. Both here
and in the United States, there have been developments towards
the use of these interviews by non-psychiatrists for population surveys. A simpler method is to use questionnaires that
involve little clinical psychiatric skill to administer.
There are now several instruments of this type including
Professor Goldberg's General Health Questionnaire (Goldberg,
1972).

The range of results that have been obtained by these more
recent methods, in spite of the fact that the techniques
themselves vary a lot, has narrowed quite considerably from
those in the earlier era. Prevalence rates for all psychiatric illness in Western urban communities have varied from
9% to approximately 20% (Wing *et al.*, 1981). Presumably the
studies that have produced the larger figures have used less
stringent criteria and the Camberwell team has given us a
useful tool for looking at this in their index of definition
(ID) that is incorporated in the PSE. This is an index of
the degree of confidence with which a specific psychiatric

diagnosis can be made and they have shown a clear relationship
between the level of confidence that is adopted and the prevalence figures obtained. If those who cannot be placed con-
fidently in any diagnostic category are excluded, the prevalence rates seem to drop to below 15%. The status of these
illness thresholds is uncertain and it is a mistake to aim
for precise prevalence figures. These are community case
rates not case rates amongst primary care attenders, though
the indications are that a fairly high proportion of community
cases do visit their GPs sometime during the illness. As a
general rule the more severe the symptoms, the more likely
the patients are to consult their doctors. Our studies in
Scotland suggest that women who have psychological symptoms
of a given severity are slightly more likely to consult than
men are with the same symptoms, though this depends on how
you do the sums and Goldberg reports a different result
(Ingham and Miller, 1981; Goldberg and Huxley, 1980).

These figures relate to patients who are well within the
range of severity shown by the majority of psychiatric
patients in hospitals and clinics. A lot of primary care
consulters do not come into the category of diagnosable
psychiatric illness and yet are experiencing emotional distress which they themselves regard as a reason for their consultation.

In one study done in a Scottish Health Centre (Ingham and
Miller, 1979), 35% of patients who had recently consulted
their doctors reported recent major threatening life events
or difficulties when they were asked, using an adaptation of
George Brown's techniques (Brown and Harris, 1978). There
was a significantly higher proportion of such people than in
a group of non-consulting controls and about a quarter of
them recognized the anxiety or depression that they were
experiencing as reasons for consulting. However, only about
50% of them were classified as ill on the "Foulds Bedford
Personal Disturbance Scale" (Foulds and Bedford, 1978). This
is a questionnaire type of scale, rather like the General
Health Questionnaire, which produces prevalence figures
fairly close to those of the standard clinical interviews
(approximately 12% in our study). The people who were
classified as ill, in addition to being emotionally distressed,
were significantly *more* likely to seek help from their doctors
than those who were distressed but not in a way that indicated
diagnosable illness. However, the actual amount of the difference was very small indeed and probably of little practical
significance. It was the severity of symptoms/distresses
that gave the best discrimination between consulters and
controls.

It may be that psychiatric illness forms a category of phenomena that differs qualitatively from normal human experience and behaviour, but that remains to be demonstrated. Even if it is true, the symptoms on which the illnesses are diagnosed certainly vary continuously from the minor distresses of everyday experience that we all suffer, through greater degrees of distress to the crippling symptoms of serious psychiatric breakdown. Whatever techniques we use for detecting cases, somewhere along the line someone has to decide on a threshold level of severity that has to be reached before any patient can be regarded as psychiatrically ill. This applies to individual symptoms as well as overall severity. There is a wide range of variation between different investigators about where this threshold should be placed. Even if a consensus is reached, however, it does seem that it will be an agreement on an arbitrary criterion. No-one has been able to make a clear statement of what we mean by illness that can be translated into an operational threshold. Ingham and Miller (1976) questioned whether the concept of prevalence should be used at all for psychiatric disorders, on the grounds that the thresholds were so arbitrary as to make the concept of illness virtually meaningless. As an alternative they suggested that comparisons of distributions of severity amongst populations of patients and non-patients conveyed all the information that was needed without any necessity for arbitrary thresholds of illness. In spite of the fact that threshold levels have now been more clearly defined in operational terms I am still inclined to that view. Prevalence can be made what you like by varying the position of the pathological threshold along the severity continuum.

The consensus threshold has settled down as one might expect, around the position that gives the best discrimination between existing psychiatric patients and the general population and this begs an important question. Patients get into the psychiatric category without anybody ever asking whether they fulfil the requirements for psychiatric illness or not. So this is very much a boot-strapping operation. We accept those who are already labelled as psychiatrically ill and use this as our criterion for illness without any closer examination. Of course there is no way of discriminating perfectly between patients and non-patients. Not only do we get roughly 15% of the general population classified as cases, but we also get approximately the same proportion of psychiatric out-patients who are false negatives and fail to reach the criterion. There is even a small group of psychiatric in-patients who are usually considered to be more severely ill, who are not sick enough to be counted as cases using the standard case finding technique. Nobody would suggest that we should now use one of the case finding instruments for clinical purposes and refuse treatment to those who do not reach the case criterion. The instruments are not infallible, but nor are the clinical decision making processes that determine whether people become psychiatric cases or not. We have no clear concept of the nature of psychiatric illness and what distinguishes it from normal psychophysiological response to stress.

It is arguable, and it is a strong argument, that there is no reason for making a distinction between the two. The doctor's job is to relieve suffering and in so doing it does not matter whether he believes he is curing some hypothetical illness or offering comfort and support to someone who is at the end of his tether in a difficult situation. It has already been indicated how we can reframe epidemiological questions in terms of a continuum from normality to abnormality and that there is no necessity to introduce hard and fast categories like *sick* and *well*. However, the distinction is important because the labels that get attached to people have an important influence on their lives. Peoples' attitudes towards those who are labelled mentally ill are substantially different from their attitudes towards those who are behaving in the same way but have not had the illness label attached to them. There are some very obvious ways in which this is so. For example you can get a week off work with a medical certificate for being ill, but not because you need a break from the boredom and frustration of doing an arduous repetitive job or because you are frightened of the boss. You can get an early retirement with full pension on grounds of ill health, but not because you are thoroughly fed up with your job and want to take it easy for the rest of your life. You can avoid being punished for an anti-social act if mental illness diminishes your responsibility for the act. Decisions of this kind that affect peoples' lives are obviously important for society but I think even more important is the fact that labelling profoundly influences attitudes including the attitudes of the person labelled towards him or herself.

Going to the doctor can be a coping device that helps people to deal with the stresses of life. Being labelled as ill, or adopting what sociologists call the sick-role, can relieve the stress. It is a legitimate excuse for not being able to meet commitments, or for behaviour that might be considered anti-social. Other people will be less demanding and more likely to exhibit solicitous and caring behaviour. Going to the doctor can be anxiety reducing and rewarding and if this happens illness behaviour is reinforced. In these circumstances, it is not in the interests of the patient to reinforce illness behaviour. When patients in this category

are recognized, we should not be saying to them "you are ill
I will give you some pills to make you better", but rather
"you are not ill, you are showing many of the symptoms and
signs that anybody would show given the stress that you are
under, I will help you to find ways of coping with your life
that are more adaptive than becoming ill".

Undoubtedly, many general practitioners recognize this type
of patient and give appropriate advice. The point is that
epidemiologists confuse the issue if they are unable to make
the distinction so that nobody knows what the prevalence
figures really mean. If the distinction between illness and
normal distress was clearer, psychiatrists and clinical
psychologists would be able to give the family doctor more
advice on how to deal with both conditions sensibly.

There is no time to go into the pros and cons of different
ways in which the term illness can be defined and it is
pointless to go in for flogging that old dead hobby horse of
some social scientists called "knocking the medical model".
But there is one definition of illness that might overcome
some of the difficulties which others engender and which
could be developed to incorporate useful guides to differential
action. It follows the concept of personal illness described
by Foulds (1976). He wrote

> When we become at least partially impaired in those
> functions which constitute us persons and when this
> impairment is sufficiently distressful to us or to
> others acting on our behalf, that means are sought
> to restore our person-hood we may be said to be
> personally ill.

The difficulty with this definition is that it includes the
seeking of means to restore. Yet people can be ill and
neither they nor anyone else do anything about it. However,
Foulds was on the right lines. The essential nature of a
personal illness is a breakdown of existing relationships
between the individual and his social environment. Modes of
adjustment and coping that have previously served to keep him
functioning within the behavioural boundaries set by the
relationships that he holds no longer work. He may virtually
cease to function or changes occur that appear as symptoms
and keep him functioning to some degree. In order to dis-
tinguish personal illness thus defined, we need to go outside
the area of symptoms and signs and to include observations of
social functioning and coping mechanisms. None of the existing case finding techniques do this and it is a major area
where research is needed for further understanding of the
natural history of psychiatric illness.

More epidemiological studies are needed in this borderline
grey area of people suffering from emotional symptoms and
signs which are not such as to be diagnosable specifically as
psychiatric illness. Sometimes they are normal responses to
circumstances, sometimes they are early indicators of psychiatric illness and they may indeed be both if stress is, as
many people think, a primary cause of psychiatric illness.
What epidemiological studies can do, particularly if they
include a longitudinal component, is to devise and validate
procedures that detect the people at greatest risk of subsequent breakdown. Once such techniques are available, the
need then will be not for further epidemiological studies
with large samples, but for intensive long-term follow-up of
small samples, even sometimes of individual cases.

We now have a fairly clear idea of the size of the problem.
In our study of health centre attenders approximately 17% of
patients admitted to having either anxiety or depression or
both and that they intended to mention the fact to the doctor.
About half of these patients were over the threshold of
personal illness on the Foulds Bedford Scale and we can be
fairly sure that others would eventually pass it if the life
stresses under which they were labouring continued. Data
from a follow-up study will shortly be available. It must
be emphasized that the Foulds Bedford Scale does not include
the observations of social functioning and coping which are
necessary for a definition of personal illness as defined
above. This is a deficiency that future research will have
to overcome.

There are already some good leads about what the risk
factors might be from the large body of research on the
effects of life events (Brown and Harris, 1978; Miller and
Ingham, 1979). We must seek methods of identifying, amongst
people who are under emotional distress, those whose coping
mechanisms and social supports are insufficient to enable
them to make adaptive positive responses to the situation.
Having identified the vulnerable group, the next aim would be
to set up a preventive service offering techniques that would
help patients to adjust their attitudes and coping strategies
in order to minimize the likelihood of breakdown. There is
no professional group with the knowledge and techniques that
fully qualifies them to offer such a service but the person
best placed to develop such knowledge and techniques is the
clinical psychologist working in primary care. Enough is
known already of the psychology of coping to enable some
well-founded guidance and help to be given (Coelho *et al.*,
1974).

Of course, this is no time to advocate the immediate
setting up of a large preventive service, even though such a

development, if soundly based, could ultimately save the health services a great deal of money. It would be fatal to set up such a service before we are in possession of the necessary know-how and can demonstrate its viability in terms of minimizing suffering and employing resources economically. The immediate need is for research aimed first at detecting those who are in greatest need of such a service, and then at developing and evaluating intervention techniques on the basis of what knowledge already exists.

To summarize, therefore, it seems that the main epidemiological problem concerning psychiatric disorder in general practice is not the detection of clearly diagnosable psychiatric illness and establishing its prevalence. It is rather the detection of patients who fall within the borderline area of emotionally distressed individuals, some of whom are coping well under the strain but others who are likely to break down. The problem is to detect those who are at greatest risk of breakdown. Our limited resources could then be devoted towards reducing the risk and maximizing the cost effectiveness of a preventive intervention programme.

REFERENCES

Bedford, A. and Foulds, G. (1978). "Delusions-Symptoms-States Inventory State of Anxiety and Depression" (Manual). N.F.E.R., Windsor, England.

Brown, G.W. and Harris, T. (1978). "Social Origins of Depression, A Study of Psychiatric Disorder in Women". Tavistock, London.

Coelho, G.V., Hamburg, D.A. and Adams, J.E. (1974). "Coping and Adaptation". Basic Books, New York.

Foulds, G.A. (1976). "The Hierarchical Nature of Personal Illness". Academic Press, London.

Goldberg, D.P. (1972). "The Detection of Psychiatric Illness by Questionnaire". Oxford University Press, London.

Goldberg, D. and Huxley, P. (1980). "Mental Illness in the Community: The Pathway to Psychiatric Care". Tavistock, London.

Ingham, J. and Miller, P. (1981). Consulting with mild symptoms in general practice. In "Recent Advances in Clinical Psychology and General Medicine (Ed. C. Main). Plenum, New York.

Ingham, J. and Miller, P.McC. (1976). The concept of prevalence applied to psychiatric disorders and symptoms. Psychological Medicine 6, 217-225.

Ingham, J. and Miller, P.McC. (1979). Symptom prevalence and severity in a general practice population. Journal of Epidemiology and Community Health 33, 3, 191-198.

Miller, P.McC. and Ingham, J.G. (1979). Reflections on the
    life-events-to illness link with some preliminary findings.
    In "Stress and Anxiety" (Eds J.G. Sarason and C.D. Spel-
    berger) 6, 313-336. John Wiley and Sons, New York.
Shepherd, M., Cooper, B., Brown, A.C. and Kalton, G.W. (1966).
    "Psychiatric Illness in General Practice". Oxford Univer-
    sity Press, London.
Spitzer, R.C. and Endicott, J. (1978). "Schedule for Affec-
    tive Disorders and Schizophrenia Life-Time Version". New
    York State Department of Mental Hygiene, New York State
    Psychiatric Institute, Biometrics Research.
Wadsworth, M. and Ingham, J. (1981). How society defines
    sickness: Illness behaviour and consultation. *In* "Founda-
    tions of Psychosomatics" (Eds M.J. Christie and P.G.
    Mellett). 341-361. John Wiley and Sons, England.
Wing, J.K., Bebbington, P. and Robins, L.N. (1981). "What is
    a Case?" Grant McIntyre Ltd., London.
Wing, J.K., Cooper, J.E. and Sartorius, N. (1974). "The
    Measurement and Classification of Psychiatric Symptoms".
    Cambridge University Press, London.

PROBLEMS OF PSYCHIATRIC CLASSIFICATION
IN GENERAL PRACTICE

Anthony W. Clare

General Practice Research Unit,
Institute of Psychiatry, De Crespigny Park,
Denmark Hill, London SE5 8AF.

For some time now the view has been expressed that the existing major classification of disease represented by the International Classification of Diseases (now in its ninth edition)
is ill-suited to the needs and realities of primary care.
This system does not have a clinical or health services
research focus and is structured so as to classify diseases
primarily according to aetiology rather than by phenomeno-
logical descriptive manifestations. This is in accord with
the historical concerns of medical statistical classification
systems starting since the time of William Farr (Israel, 1978).
These systems have been structured to group diseases by ana-
tomical site and to facilitate the vital statistics function
of recording causes of death. Hence the strength of the
current ICD classificatory system is that it promotes an
aetiologically oriented approach to clinical diagnosis and
the pathological descriptions of causes of death and morbidity.
However, in consequence, it is criticized for failing to provide clinicians with a useful tool for describing the mix of
physical, mental and social symptoms and problems for which a
unitary aetiologically-based diagnosis is either inappropriate
or impossible (Shepherd *et al.*, 1966; Regier *et al.*, 1982).
   Major modifications to ICD have occurred in attempts to
facilitate more clinical and descriptive approaches to classification in primary care. In 1958 a report of studies conducted by the then College of General Practitioners demonstrated that almost half the problems brought to family
physicians could not be assigned a "diagnosis", at least at
the initial visit, that was compatible with the edition of
ICD that was available at that time. Over the next few years
a group of the College's members evolved a classification of

symptoms, complaints, conditions, problems and reasons for
seeking help that appeared to be more appropriate to the array
of perceived illness and problems of living that constitute
the burden of suffering at this level of intervention (College
of General Practitioners, 1959; 1963). This new classification was materially different both in concept and terminology
from the traditional ICD and over the next few years it was
refined and tested. After further modifications, a version
became formalized as the International Classification of
Health Problems in Primary Care (ICHPPC) by the Classification
Committee of the World Organization of National Colleges,
Academies and Academic Associations of General Practitioners/
Family Physicians (WONCA) and the US clinical modification of
the ICD-9, entitled the ICD-9 CM. An even more radical change
in the framework for classification of general practice
problems is the recently developed Reason for Visit (RVC)
classification (Schneider *et al.*, 1979) used in the US National
Ambulatory Medical Care Survey. The RVC is intended to serve
a separate function from the ICD diagnoses and to exist as a
parallel classification system for recording the patient's
"diagnosis" as opposed to the physician's diagnosis of the
reason for visit. Major objectives of this classification
are to identify why patients use the health care system and
to assist in determining the relative role of self-care,
family care and professional care (both primary and specialized) in meeting patient needs.

However, none of these classifications produce statistics
relating to psychological morbidity and social problems which
are congruent with statistics produced in the course of in-
depth research into incidence and prevalence in primary care.
The first and second national morbidity surveys in the United
Kingdom, which relied on ICD diagnostic categories, and the
NAMCS study in the United States reported relatively low rates
(less than 5% of all diagnoses made) of recorded mental disorder diagnoses while the use of ICHPPC (Wood *et al.*, 1975)
resulted in even lower rates. The lack of a more appropriate
classificatory and recording system has serious implications
for proposed large-scale surveys of primary care such as the
planned third National Morbidity Survey.

In contrast, more detailed examinations of patients in
general practice settings by means of standardized psychiatric
assessments or patient self-reporting questionnaires have con-
sistently revealed that there is a substantially greater
number of patients with mental disorders and a large degree
of psychosocial morbidity which is neither recognized in GP
survey studies nor reported in medical records (Shepherd *et
al.*, 1966; Rawnsley, 1966; Stoller and Krupinski, 1969; Goldberg and Blackwell, 1970; Wood *et al.*, 1975; Hoeper *et al.*,

1979). More systematic data collecting and recording in primary care confirms the research finding that the proportion of the total morbidity pool which is made up of psychiatric disorders classifiable in terms of ICD diagnoses is in excess of 12% (Morrell, 1971; Morrell et al., 1970).

This prevalence estimate appears true in the developing parts of the world too (Mbanefo, 1971; Harding, 1973; Giel and Van Luijk, 1979; Ndetei and Muhangi, 1979). Such studies, however, are of necessity rather small and potentially unrepresentative. However, the recently completed WHO Collaborative Study on Strategies for Extending Mental Health Care, using relatively stringent criteria to establish the presence of psychiatric morbidity, found an overall prevalence of just under 14% in over 1600 patients attending primary health facilities in 4 developing countries (Harding et al., 1980).

The results of these and other studies suggest that the routine recording of ICD Section V (Mental Disorders) and Section XVI (Symptoms and Ill-defined Conditions) tends to under-represent the prevalence rates for mental disorders and other psychosocial problems. One solution to this problem that has recently been proposed (WHO, 1979; Regier et al., 1982) is that there should be a triaxial approach adopted with regard to the classification of primary care problems, with one axis provided for the recording of physical disorders, a second axis for the recording to psychological symptoms and syndromes and a third for the recording of social problems. Such a multi-axial approach, it is argued, would clearly emphasize the role of the primary care physician in the identification and management of significant social as well as psychological disturbance. Such a multi-axial classificatory system would possess the added advantage of providing data relating to the vexed question of the relationship between psychosocial problems and all forms of medical diagnoses, including physical, which are currently made in primary care.

In the face of wide discrepancies between the routinely recorded diagnoses and rates obtained from direct surveys of primary care practices, one is forced to re-examine both the recording practices and the current classification system. Medical records which inaccurately record the presence of a mental disorder or social problem have a markedly reduced utility for patient care, for the monitoring of the quality of that care and for providing the data base for the planning of needed services. There is reason too to suspect that the framework provided by a classification of physical, mental and social disturbance which, as in the case of the ICD, is heavily biased towards the organic end of the disorder spectrum may have a major impact on physicians' expectations of their professional role.

In addition to shortcomings in the classification of health
problems in primary care, an important contributory factor to
the variation between prevalence findings is differences
between individual general practitioners in their ability to
identify psychological and social problems in their patients.
Shepherd and his colleagues reported that over half the non-
random variance in reporting of psychiatric problems by
general practitioners "must be ascribed largely to differences
between doctors rather than between practice populations
(Shepherd *et al.*, 1966). Goldberg and his colleagues have
argued that the ability of the individual general practitioner
to make accurate assessments "is related to personality
variables and interview style" (Goldberg, 1980). Goldberg
and his colleagues have reported that a research psychiatrist
was significantly superior to general practitioners in his
ability to identify symptomatic patients as "ill" (Marks *et
al.*, 1979) but the correlations between his ratings of the
severity of patients' disturbances with their own self-ratings
were no higher than those obtained by the general practitioners
he was observing. It is not clear from this study the extent
to which the availability of background and stored information to the general practitioners affected the weighting they
placed on the significance of expressed symptoms. Before con-
cluding that general practitioners are seriously deficient in
their ability to detect psychiatric morbidity in their
patients, it is necessary to be absolutely clear as to the
notions of psychiatric "caseness" which such general practitioners hold. That caution needs to be exercised in interpreting the apparently haphazard behaviour of GPs is confirmed
by Raynes' detailed study of the consultations of 10 general
practitioners (Raynes, 1979). Her findings supported Howie's
view that much of what appears to be haphazard drug prescribing in primary care can be explained if it is understood that
the treatment of "symptoms" constitutes a large part of
primary care and that treatment more often than not follows
not from diagnosis but from the identification and the explora-
tion of signs (Howie, 1972). However, as Raynes points out,
the identification of signs and the eliciting of symptoms by
general practitioners are still poorly understood. Such
attempts to clarify the picture have tended to rely on comparisons of the performance of the general practitioner with the
results of a self-report symptom questionnaire (Goldberg and
Blackwell, 1970) or the diagnostic decisions of a research
psychiatrist (Marks *et al.*, 1979). To date, there has been
no systematic study which has examined the kinds of variation
and disagreement which occur when general practitioners are
presented with the same patient and are asked to make a diagnosis and plan treatment although there have been a number of

ingenious attempts to mimic the clinical situation for research
purposes (Howie, 1972).

For the purposes of experimental study, the factors which
lead to diagreements and difficulties of communication in this
area can be regarded as deriving from 3 principal sources:

1. variations at the level of observation and perception;
2. variations in the inference drawn from such observations;
and
3. variations in the nosological schemata employed by the
   individual clinician.

These 3 sources of variation are open to investigation.
Indeed, a research strategy based on an analysis of these 3
sources of error has already been applied in at least one
experimental approach to psychiatric diagnosis in a specialized psychiatric setting (Shepherd *et al.*, 1968). It would
seem that here is a potentially fruitful area for collaborative research involving general practitioners and psychiatrists.

To contemplate some of the fundamental issues in developing
a workable strategy however, we must first separate the 2
different intellectual activities that are involved in procedures of classification (Feinstein, 1978). The first is
taxonomic. It consists of demarcating, defining or otherwise
establishing the categories that will be used for diagnosis.
The second procedure is *diagnostic* and consists of providing
rules of identification, enabling the selection of categories
pertinent to a particular person. Taxonomy, as Feinstein has
recently reminded us, consists of providing definitions but
diagnosis requires operational identification (Feinstein,
1978). In the area of primary care, both taxonomic and diagnostic considerations are involved in any attempt to clarify
classification in primary care. The most prominent problems
of psycho-social nosology in this setting are:

1. the absence of operational criteria and standardization for
   designating basic elements of observed "evidence" which,
   in this setting, include such symptoms as anxiety, depression, tension, tiredness, etc. The major attempts in
   psychiatry to develop an acceptable classification, such
   as the PSE (Wing *et al.*, 1974) and the DSM-111 (Spitzer *et
   al.*, 1976) have been concerned with what is done after
   these basic elements have been designated but there have
   been no attempts to bring consistency and uniformity to
   the basic designations themselves. Such terms as *anxiety*,
   depression and *tension* are in themselves miniature diagnoses (Feinstein, 1978), particularly for the general
   practitioner, but in the absence of operational criteria

we have no idea of the extent to which general practitioners
differ in their conceptualizations of such "diagnoses" nor
in the inferences they draw from perceiving such symptoms
to be present;
2. the difficulty of external validation given the current
absence of correlations either with aetiologic evidence or
with data for prognosis.

Taking the second problem first, the easiest form of
external validation is to use prognosis and therapy but in the
primary care setting there is a paucity of evidence concerning
the natural history of the "diseases" in question and we know
far less about the efficacy of the treatments of psychosocial
disorders in general practice than is often appreciated. The
absence of operational criteria and standardization in relation
to such symptoms as anxiety and depression contribute to the
difficulties of identifying and treating them. The argument
over the classification of depression, for example, is hardly
an academic one. It is worth noting, for example, that general
practitioners are readily and regularly criticized for their
apparent misuse of the 2 classes of psychotropic drugs defined
as anti-depressants and anxiolytics. A number of observers
have drawn attention to the tendency of general practitioners
to use subtherapeutic doses of antidepressants (Johnson, 1974;
Tyrer, 1978), to use antidepressants and anxiolytics inter-
changeably and arbitrarily (Weissman and Klerman, 1977;
Weissman, 1981) and to achieve dispiritingly low levels of
drug compliance on the part of their patients (Johnson, 1980).
General practitioners are perfectly justified in questioning the assumption, often explicit in the utterances of critical psychiatrists, that the depressions and the anxieties
presenting in general practice and community settings are
identical to those familiar to psychiatrists. Current research
does suggest that the majority of psychiatric disorders presenting in primary care and identified in community surveys
will fall within a single broad diagnostic category - depression with or without associated anxiety. But that is as far
as agreement goes. The questions then appear as numerous as
they are complex. Are there 2 types of depression, the one,
psychotic and endogenous, the other neurotic or reactive?
Are there 2 equally distinct groups of patients, the one
suffering from psychotic depression, being relatively small
numerically but important in terms of severity of symptomat-
ology and outcome, the other larger, more heterogeneous
suffering from neurotic depression? Summarizing a very broad
literature there is general agreement (Kendell, 1976) that
there are indeed 2 kinds of depression and that there is a
distinct group of patients suffering from the disease entity

of psychotic depression. But there is no general agreement
as to the distribution of neurotic depression. Garside (1981)
suggests that neurotic depression is probably best regarded
as continuous rather than bimodal at least until shown to be
otherwise. On the basis of such a view, he goes on to make
the potentially useful suggestion that the attempt to arrive
at a differential diagnosis in relation to depressed patients
is inappropriate. It is not a case of asking "Is this patient
suffering from psychotic or neurotic depression?" a question
resting on the assumption that each is categorically distinct
from the other. Rather, 2 separate questions should be asked:
first, is the patient suffering from psychotic depression or
is he not; and second, to what extent is he suffering from
neurotic depression.

Garside's suggestion has interesting implications for the
argument concerning the prescription of psychotropic drugs.
There is an assumption that antidepressants are indicated in
the treatment of psychotic depression but may have much less
to offer in non-psychotic depressions. Clinically, such a
picture can further be clouded by the co-existence of anxiety.
Many general practitioners appear to use anxiolytics and or
sub-optimal doses of antidepressants largely for sedative
purposes in patients who appear primarily anxious or whose
depressed mood is strongly contaminated by features of anxiety.
In a study undertaken by the General Practice Research Unit
we found that whereas men who complained mainly of depression
invariably received an antidepressant, women who so complained
were as likely to receive an anxiolytic as an antidepressant
(Clare and Williams, 1981). When anxiety was judged to be
the main complaint, an anxiolytic was almost invariably prescribed for both men and women. As against that, the presence
of anxiety in the setting of depression may be less significant
from the point of drug therapy than GPs have been trained to
think. Johnstone and her co-workers (Johnstone *et al.*, 1980)
were unable to divide a sample of 240 neurotic outpatients
into anxious and depressed groups on the basis of the clinical
picture. Nor did it appear to matter very much in that the
outcome appeared to be good regardless of medication. These
authors were moved to conclude that the distinction between
anxiety and depression in neurotic outpatients "is of no
practical value with regard to drug treatment" although they
did add that if psychotropic drugs have to be given tricyclic
antidepressants appear more likely to be effective than benzodiazepines. A WHO collaborative, multi-centred study on the
assessment of depressive disorders also confirmed the difficulty of distinguishing anxiety from depressive states, noting
that "anxiety and depression appear among the most common
symptoms of depression in all centres" a finding which casts

doubt on the validity of the separation of a subtype of
"anxious depression" (Jablensky *et al.*, 1981).

So how is the general practitioner to detect the relatively
few patients suffering from psychotic depression with or without neurotic features including anxiety from the many neuroti-
cally depressed presenting to him? Much of the evidence we
need is derived from studies based on hospital and clinic
populations. It has, however, been suggested that the presence
of psychomotor retardation or agitation, lack of reactivity to
environmental changes, severe depressed mood, depressive
delusions, self-reproach and loss of interest in pleasurable
activity are symptoms distinctive for endogenous/psychotic
depression (Nelson and Charney, 1981). Sleep disturbance,
suicidal feelings, weight and appetite loss, on the other
hand, are not useful differentiating complaints. How many
endogenously depressed patients a general practitioner will
encounter in the course of a year is unclear, but such data
as exist suggest that the number is likely to be small. Does
this mean that prescribing tricyclic antidepressant medication for the very much larger number of non-endogenously
depressed patients is inappropriate? Again, without information derived from general practice studies concerning the
efficacy of antidepressants, anxiolytics and non-drug interventions, it is difficult to be dogmatic.

An essential aspect of any classification is that it should
be clinically useful. Categorization should, for example,
suggest the most appropriate intervention. Feinstein's
advice to psychiatrists interested in classification that they
should concentrate on the "raw evidence" and on "standardization of the elements of evidence" (Feinstein, 1978) is applicable to general practitioners too. But even to begin,
general practitioners are going to have to subject to greater
scrutiny the diagnostic terminology and the systems of classification which they do employ.

REFERENCES

Clare, A. and Williams, P. (1981). Factors leading to psycho-
    tropic drug prescription. *In* "The Misuse of Psychotropic
    Drugs", Chap. 17, 83-86. Gaskell Books, London.
College of General Practitioners Research Committee of Council
    (1963). A classification of disease. (Amended version).
    Journal of the Royal College of General Practitioners **6**,
    207-216.
Feinstein, A.R. (1978). A critical overview of diagnosis in
    psychiatry. *In* "Psychiatric Diagnosis" (Eds V.M. Rakoff,
    H.C. Stancer and H.B. Kedward), Chap. 9, 189-206. Macmillan,
    London.

Garside, R.F. (1981). Bimodality and the nature of depression. *British Journal of Psychiatry* **139**, 168-169.

Giel, R. and Van Luijk, V.N. (1979). Psychiatric morbidity in a small Ethiopian town. *British Journal of Psychiatry* **115**, 149-162.

Goldberg, D. (1980). Training of family physicians in mental health skills: implications of recent research. *In* "Mental Health Services In Primary Care Settings", Conference Report, April 2-3, 1979, Mental Health Service System Reports. Series DN No. 2. U.S. Department of Health and Human Services, N.I.M.H. Rockville, Maryland, 20857.

Goldberg, D.P. and Blackwell, B. (1970). Psychiatric illness in general practice: A detailed study using a new method of case identification. *British Medical Journal* **2**, 439-443.

Harding, T. (1973). The detection of psychiatric illness by questionnaire in Jamaica. *West Indian Medical Journal* **22**, 190-191.

Harding, T.W., De Arango, M.V., Baltazar, J., Climent, C.E., Ibrahim, H.H.A., Ladrigo-Ignacio, L., Stinivasa Murthy, R. and Wig, N.N. (1980). Mental disorders in primary health care: A study of their frequency and diagnosis in four developing countries. *Psychological Medicine* **10**, 231-241.

Hoeper, E.W., Greg, R., Cleary, P.D., Regier, D.A. and Goldberg, I.D. (1979). Estimated prevalence of RDC mental disorder in primary medical care. *International Journal of Mental Health* **8**, 2, 8-15.

Howie, J.G.R. (1972). Diagnosis - the Achilles heel? *Journal of the Royal College of General Practitioners* **22**, 310-315.

International Classification of Health Problems in Primary Care. (ICHPPC-2), 2nd edition. 1979 Revision. Oxford University Press, London.

Israel, R.A. (1978). The international classification of diseases: Two hundred years of development. *Public Health Reports* **93**, 2, 150-152.

Jablensky, A., Sartorius, N., Gulbinat, W. and Ernberg, G. (1981). Characteristics of depressive patients contacting psychiatric services in four cultures. *Acta Psychiatrica Scandinavica* **63**, 367-383.

Johnson, D.A.W. (1974). A study of the use of antidepressant medication in general practice. *British Journal of Psychiatry* **125**, 186-192.

Johnstone, E.C., Cunningham Owens, D.G., Frith, C.D., McPherson, K., Dowie, C., Riley, G. and Gold, A. (1980). Neurotic illness and its response to anxiolytic and antidepressant treatment. *Psychological Medicine* **10**, 321-328.

Kendell, R.E. (1976). The classification of depression: a review of contemporary confusion. *British Journal of Psychiatry* **129**, 15-28.

Marks, J.N., Goldberg, D. and Hillier, V. (1979). Determinants of the ability of general practitioners to detect psychiatric illness. *Psychological Medicine* **9**, 2, 337-353.

Mbanefo, S.E. (1971). The general practitioner and psychiatry. *In* "Psychiatry and Mental Health Care in General Practice" (Ed. A. Boroffka), 45-49. University of Ibadan, Ibadan.

Morrell, D.C., Gage, H.G. and Robinson, N.A. (1970). Patterns of demand in general practice. *Journal of the Royal College of General Practitioners* **19**, 331.

Morrell, D.C. (1971). Expressions of morbidity in general practice. *British Medical Journal* **ii**, 454.

Nelson, J.C. and Charney, D.S. (1981). The symptoms of major depressive illness. *American Journal of Psychiatry* **138**, 1-13.

Noletei, D.M. and Muhangi, J. (1979). The prevalence and clinical presentation of psychiatric illness in a rural setting in Kenya. *British Journal of Psychiatry* **135**, 269-272.

Rawnsley, K. (1966). Congruence of independent measures of psychiatric morbidity. *Journal of Psychosomatic Research* **10**, 84-93.

Raynes, N.V. (1979). Factors affecting the prescribing of psychotropic drugs in general practice consultations. *Psychological Medicine* **9**, 671-679.

Regier, D.A., Burns, B.J., Burke, J.D., Clare, A., Lipkin, M., Spitzer, R., Wood, M., Gulbinat, W. and Williams, J.B.W. (1982). Proposed classification of social problems and psychological symptoms for inclusion in a Classification of Health Problems. *In* "Psychosocial Factors Affecting Health", (Eds M. Lipkin, W. Gulbinat and K. Kupka), Praeger, New York. In press.

Research Committee of the College of General Practitioners (1959). A classification of disease. *Journal of the College of General Practitioners* **2**, 140-159.

Schneider, D., Aplleton, L. and McLemore, T. (1979). A reason for visit classification for ambulatory care. *In* "Vital and Health Statistics", Series 2, No. 78, DHEW Pub. No. (PHS) 78-1352. Public Health Service, Hyattsville, Maryland 20782.

Shepherd, M., Cooper, B., Brown, A.C. and Kalton, G.W. (1966). "Psychiatric Illness in General Practice". Oxford University Press, London.

Shepherd, M., Brooke, E.M., Cooper, J.E. and Lin, T.Y. (1968). An experimental approach to psychiatric diagnosis. *In* "Acta Psychiatrica Scandinavica", Suppl. 201, Vol. 44, Munksgaard, Copenhagen.

Spitzer, R.L., Endicott, J. and Robbins, E. (1976). Clinical criteria for psychiatric diagnosis and DSM-III. *American Journal of Psychiatry* **132**, 11, 1187-1192.

Stoller, A. and Krupinski, J. (1969). Psychiatric disturbances. *In* "Report on a National Morbidity Survey", 48, N.H.M.R.C. Canberra.

Tyrer, P. (1978). Drug treatment of psychiatric patients in general practice. *British Medical Journal* **2**, 1008-1010.

Weissman, M.M. (1981). Depression and its treatment in a U.S. urban community. *Archives of General Psychiatry* **38**, 417-421.

Weissman, M.M. and Klerman, G.L. (1977). The chronic depressive in the community. Unrecognized and poorly treated. *Comprehensive Psychiatry* **18**, 523-532.

Wing, J.K., Cooper, J.E. and Sartorius, N. (1974). "The Description and Classification of Psychiatric Symptoms: An Instruction Manual for the PSE and CATEGO system". Cambridge University Press, London.

World Health Organization. (1979). "Recording Health Problems Tri-axially". An International Collaborative Study Proposed by the WHO, Geneva.

World Health Organization. (1981). "Recording Health Problems Tri-axially: the Physical, Psychological and Social Components of Primary Health Care Contacts". 1st Meeting of Investigators Collaborating in the WHO-co-ordinated Project. Bellagio, Italy, February 9-13.

Wood, M., Mayo, F. and Marsland, D. (1975). A systems approach to patient care, curriculum and research in family practice. *Journal of Medical Education* **50**, 1106-1112.

APPENDIX
GENERAL PRACTICE CONSULTATION
VIDEO EXERCISE

Anthony W. Clare and Karl Sabbagh*

*General Practice Research Unit,
Institute of Psychiatry, De Crespigny Park,
Denmark Hill, London SE5 8AF*

**MSD Foundation, Tavistock House,
Tavistock Square, London WC1H 9LG.*

A video recording of a general practice consultation was shown to the conference participants. The recording, prepared by the MSD Foundation, consisted of a 10 minute interview between a male general practitioner and a 44 year old married woman.

Mrs M., who had not attended this doctor before, came because for about one week she had been feeling " a bit run down", "tired" and "depressed". Normally, on her own account, she was a very energetic, busy and competent woman. She had 11 children, 9 by her first husband, and 2 by her second. In addition to looking after the youngest 2 children, she worked as a part-time cashier. In the course of the interview, a number of items relating to her previous history emerged. Eleven years before, her first marriage broke up and she became very distressed and cut her wrist. She spent a period of time in a psychiatric hospital. Following the birth of her 11th child she underwent a hysterectomy for fibroids, since when she complained of discomfort and occasional pain when passing urine. Three months prior to this consultation, she had been presribed stimulants for weight reduction by one of the GP's partners but had discontinued taking these for about one month.

Further questioning by the GP revealed that Mrs M. felt more tired and lacking in energy than truly depressed, that she found difficulty relaxing and that she herself was not clear why she was feeling like this. She said her second marriage was happy and that she normally enjoyed her work. Towards the end of the interview, the GP elicited the fact that one of the 2 children, a son by her second husband was an albino. The GP suggested a MSU, in view of the abdominal discomfort, a follow-up appointment in a week and a similar period of rest. The possibility that her symptoms might be a reaction to the discontinuation of the weight-reducing tablets was also raised.

Each conference participant was then asked to answer 3 questions relating to what he/she had just seen:

1. How would you define this patient's problem?
2. What action would you take?
3. Do you feel this GP handled the consultation well?

RESULTS

One hundred and thirty six participants replied to the 3 questions. Fifty nine were general practitioners, 38 were psychiatrists, 12 were psychologists, 7 were social workers, 5 were sociologists, and the remaining 15 included a probation officer, a health visitor, 2 counsellors, 2 community physicians, 2 community psychiatric nurses, 2 civil servants, 2 medical journalists and 2 lay people. In this brief report, only the responses of the GPs and the psychiatrists will be considered.

1. Definition of the Problem

In the light of the opinion widely expressed at the conference that the making of a formal diagnosis in general practice is more the exception than the rule, it is interesting to note (Table 1) that 40% of the GP respondents and 45% of the psychiatrists were prepared to select a definite diagnosis in this case. Depression was a popular choice but whereas psychiatrists also opted for a diagnosis of a mixed anxiety-depression neurosis, GPs favoured anxiety state as an alternative.

Many of those reluctant to make a diagnosis emphasized the lack of information concerning the underlying nature of the patient's problem and the complicated mixture of social (work and family), physical (abdominal pain and dysuria) and psychological (fatigue, depression) problems presented.

CLARE and SABBAGH

TABLE 1

GP and psychiatrists' definition of problem

Diagnosis	GPs		Psychiatrists	
None made	18 (30%)		16 (42%)	
Tenative Dx. suggested	18 (30%)		5 (13%)	
Definite Dx. made	23 (40%)		17 (45%)	
	Depression	11	Depression	8
	Anxiety	10	Mixed	8
	Mixed	1	Anxiety	1
	Other	1		

TABLE 2

Action recommended by GPs and psychiatrists

Action	GPs	Psychiatrists
Psychotropic drug	3 (3.7%)	1 (2%)
Reassurance, wait and see	26 (31.7%)	12 (22.2%)
Full history and mental state examination	25 (30.5%)	15 (27.2%)
Physical examination	14 (17%)	8 (15%)
Family interview	5 (6%)	7 (13%)
Involvement of other professionals (SW, HV, etc.)	6 (7.4%)	4 (7.5%)
Involvement of psychiatrist	0 —	3 (5.6%)
Drugs possibly in the future	3 (3.7%)	4 (7.5%)

Those who were prepared to make an unequivocal diagnosis
appeared in the main to be using the diagnostic term des-
criptively, that is to say they did not seem to see it as
having prescriptive implications to judge by their responses
to the second question.

2. Action to be Taken

Only 3 GPs and 1 psychiatrist felt that psychotropic drugs
were indicated on the basis of the consultation, although 3
more GPs and 4 psychiatrists expressed the view that such
drugs might well be needed after clarification of the patient's
problem. In the main, however, the respondents favoured the
course adopted by the GP but many did express the view that
a more thorough assessment including a more detailed history
was needed (Table 2).
     There was no clear-cut relationship between whether a
formal diagnosis was made or not and any particular course of
action chosen. In general, the GPs and psychiatrists were in
agreement but some respondents' comments revealed sharp differences. One psychiatrist believed that the GP would need
to discuss the case "with someone with dynamic psychiatric
understanding", while several other psychiatrists suggested
family therapy. Those GPs who favoured involving other
family members did so on account of the advantages to be
anticipated in terms of obtaining further information rather
than for any therapeutic reason.

3. GP's Handling of Consultation

The replies to this question did reveal differences between
the GPs and the psychiatrists. Twice as many psychiatrists
proportionately than GPs disapproved of the general practitioner's handling of the consultation. More of the GPs
qualified their approval with comments whereas the psychiatrists tended to approve or disapprove with less qualification
(Table 3). One in 3 of the psychiatrists considered the
interview to have been handled badly and many expressed this
view with force. One psychiatrist, known for his work alongside GPs in primary care, declared that the GP was "a kindly
doctor wanting to help but seriously handicapped by lack of
training in techniques for interviewing a fairly typical
psychologically disturbed patient in general practice" while
a Professor of psychiatry commented dismissively that the GP
had done little more "than a sympathetic layman could".
Another declared that the video illustrated "the usual myth
of the GP who knows his patient" while a fourth commented
that he had made poor use of his time and "was clearly showing

TABLE 3

Opinion of GP's handling of the consultation

	Approval	Approval with qualification	Disapproval
GPs	29 (49%)	21 (36%)	9 (15%)
Psychiatrists	16 (42%)	10 (26%)	12 (32%)

off his interview technique as well as indulging in a number of histrionic non-verbal mannerisms". Other psychiatrists, however, regarded the interview as sympathetic, empathic and warm, congratulated the GP on his skillful use of the available time and expressed satisfaction that he had avoided the use of technical terms and the prescription pad. Those who expressed qualified approval mentioned the need for a fuller investigation of the patient's psychological and social circumstances and a detailed physical examination.

The GPs were somewhat less critical of their colleague's performance although several did feel that he had appeared bored, had left the patient dissatisfied, had placed too much emphasis on physical factors (e.g. the weight-reducing tablets) and had insufficiently explored the patient's psychological problems and social circumstances. Many, while generally approving of the GP's handling, felt he could have been more active in his questioning, could, for example, have asked the patient what it was she wanted of him, and could have given her clearer details of his future plans concerning her management. GPs who disapproved of the consultation tended to criticize the doctor's manner, his "helplessness", his unconvincing "explanation" (the possible role of the weight-reducing tablets) and his alleged failure to make "supportive" comments.

DISCUSSION

The video exercise helped to focus the conference participants' attention on the actual realities of the general practice consultation and, to that extent, it served a useful purpose. However, it also illustrated the complexity of the issues involved. The ill-formed nature of many psychological symptoms presented in general practice was neatly exemplified in the consultation in question, a fairly typical consultation it should be said, and the extent to which doctors, even in primary care, are often dependent on the quality of medical notes, was once again shown. Perhaps the most striking finding, however, was the lack of unanimity concerning the GP's handling of the consultation. The GP, a very experienced man and active in the education of GP trainees, was variously seen as excellent, skilled, reassuring and supportive, and as incompetent, bored and disorganized. Psychiatrists, in particular, were forthright in the criticisms and the 3 who saw a possible role for psychiatry in the management of such a case all pointed to the apparent need for a proper psychiatric examination in elucidating the underlying problem.

FOLLOW-UP VIDEO

After the respondents had completed their forms, Dr Clare then showed a video recording of an interview he had conducted with Mrs M. 1 year after the consultation with the GP had taken place.

Mrs M. described a follow-up interview with the GP 1 week later in which she had discussed in more detail her anxieties about her albino son who was being bullied and teased in his school. She had been impressed by her GP's remarks implying that she might be overdoing things and had taken a week off work which resulted in her being declared redundant. However, she decided not to seek another job but to involve herself with her own family, the older members of which lived locally. She had become particularly involved with a 17 year old daughter who was having recurrent personal problems, had made numerous suicidal attempts, had been a psychiatric in-patient on a number of occasions and was currently on psychiatric medication. Mrs M. expressed doubts about the usefulness of such medication and had been grateful that her GP had not prescribed anything for her.

Mrs M. also described how the symptoms she experienced when she visited her GP had been different from and less severe than the symptoms she experienced at the time of her marital break-up and her psychiatric admission 11 years previously.

Finally, Mrs M. commented on how valuable she had found the original interview with her GP, how she would return to him were she ever to have any further emotional or social problems (while being content to see one of his partners for less important matters, such as physical ill-health!) and how being able to talk about her worries over her son, even though little

practical changes could be effected, had been immensely
reassuring. She now felt more confident re her son,
and he did seem to be coping a little better too. She
was quite certain that within a short time of having
first seen her GP she had felt very much better and was
now in excellent health.

ACKNOWLEDGEMENTS

The authors wish to express their grateful appreciation to
Mrs M. for her generous co-operation and to the general practitioner involved who consented readily to his consultation
being shown to a multi-disciplinary audience. We are grateful too for the co-operation of the MSD Foundation in recording the original consultation and in organizing and recording
the follow-up interview. The assistance of Peter Joyce of
the Institute of Psychiatry in showing the recordings at
Oxford is also acknowledged with thanks.

SESSION 1
DISCUSSION

Dr Peter TOMSON (Abbots Langley): Dr Ingham suggested that
practitioners might get seriously involved in some form of
intervention when people encountered stress. In our Report,
"The Prevention of Psychiatric Disorders in General Practice"
we stated that we would only want to be actively involved with
those who were at risk for other reasons, whether historical,
e.g. the death of their mother, or social in terms of poor
housing. We would not recommend that every bereaved person
would warrant a special intervention.

Dr INGHAM: I agree with you. I was not implying that some
preventive measures, for example in cases of bereavement, that
are certainly within the scope of general practitioners, should
be done routinely, but I am concerned about widening this to
many stressful life circumstances when not enough is known to
identify the most vulnerable people.

Dr N. MISRA (Treorchy): How can a general practitioner like
myself identify that a person with emotional disturbance can
still cope? Because if he cannot then I must give preventive
counselling or whatever?

Dr INGHAM: I can only give you limited advice here. Find
out how the person coped with past problems. You can then
judge whether this is a coping person or a non-coping person.
Of course, if he is a new patient it is more difficult.

Dr Brendan KELLY (Merthyr Tydfil): I work as a general practitioner in Merthyr Tydfil. In that town we have a multi-
disciplinary unit for prophylactic intervention. It is housed
in an old manor house and staffed by 4 psychiatrists, one
psychologist, one general practitioner, 4 nurses and 3 social
workers. People who feel the need of help, who have difficulties in adjusting or full-scale psychiatric disorders, can
come either on their own or be referred by a neighbour or a
friend or a relative or by their GP; it seems to be working.

Mrs June LAIT (Swansea): I was very impressed by Dr Ingham's advice to doctors and all concerned with medicine not to set up a full-scale preventive service until there was some prospect of it being effective. One weakness in this field is the lack of rigorous assessment of whether these hopeful ventures are succeeding and of the criteria which will determine that success. The danger is of raising expectations in patients that you can make them happy. You must inform people what you cannot do and reduce their inordinate expectations of you.

The CHAIRMAN: Thank you. That seems to me a most important point.

Dr Derek RICHTER (Tadworth): In defining our problems could I draw attention to the great inequality in the handling by GPs of psychiatric patients, especially chronic patients returning to the community. Some GPs deal very well with these patients, understanding them, getting them to go back on their drugs, establishing good relations with the psychiatrist or the social worker and altogether helping the patient to cope and to continue living and working in the community. But some GPs cannot achieve that understanding and help. Is this a matter of training?

The CHAIRMAN: I wish it were only a question of training. It is easy to answer that such GPs should refer those cases to somebody more skilled and more interested but, if they do not recognize them, you have an additional block.

Dr MISRA (Treorchy): Is the classification Dr Clare was suggesting different from that used by general practitioners or is it inadequate for general practitioners to use?

Dr Anthony CLARE: Classifications currently familiar to GPs are, in general inadequate and are poorly used. It is not clear whether by tinkering with a uni-axial classification you could devise a better system for reporting on the problems in primary care. Why not have a classification system that reflects the intricacy of problems as they present to the GP so that he can report what he finds - namely a multi-axial classification reflecting the physical, psychological and social mix? The GP is under great pressure from psychiatrists, drug companies and others who claim he is missing serious psychiatric illness. How is he to identify the unknown number, usually assumed to be relatively small, of patients suffering from serious biological, i.e. endogenous, depression from the large pool of "depressive morbidity" that presents to him? If he prescribes antidepressants widely he is criticized but if he restricts his practice he is under attack by clinical psychiatrists for missing serious and suicidal patients who may destroy themselves. That is still a very lively issue.

THE RECOGNITION OF PSYCHOLOGICAL ILLNESS BY GENERAL PRACTITIONERS

David Goldberg

*Department of Psychiatry,
The University Hospital of South Manchester,
West Didsbury, Manchester M20 8LR.*

General practitioners vary widely between themselves in their ability to recognize psychological illness among their patients. Michael Shepherd and his colleagues were among the first to draw attention to the wide variations between London GPs in the *level* of psychiatric illness they reported. Some doctors reported psychiatric consulting rates as low as 38 per 1000 at risk, while others reported rates as high as 323 per 1000 at risk. There is a ninefold difference between these rates. The researchers used a psychiatric screening questionnaire in 14 of the practices in an attempt to discover the extent to which these differences were due to true differences in prevalence between the practices, and found no relationship between the level of illness predicted by the questionnaire, and the level reported by the doctor.

Only two factors were found which related to whether a doctor reported high levels of psychiatric morbidity: one relating to the doctor's attitudes, and the other to his practice. Those who thought psychological factors were important in the aetiology of various diseases tended to report high levels, as did those who had many patients entering and leaving their practice lists over the course of a year. I was able to extend these observations during a year spent observing family doctors in Philadelphia, USA. Doctors who worked long hours reported higher rates than those who worked short hours, and high status doctors (those with the MD degree, with hospital affiliations and members of the AMA) reported lower rates than low status doctors (osteopaths, and those without hospital attachments and professional affiliations). In a later study in Manchester we confirmed that the doctors who thought psychological factors were important in the aetiology of physical disease tended to have high rates of ascertainment of psychiatric disorder.

So far so good. We have so far dealt with the level of
psychiatric disorder reported - and such levels will presumably be related to the threshold used for case identification.
Some doctors will only regard floridly psychotic patients as
"psychiatric", while others will include very minor, transient
disorders in their concept of a "case". The former will
report low rates, and the latter high.

However, knowing the *level* of morbidity reported by a given
doctor tells us nothing about his accuracy as a case detector.
Two doctors may each report a level of 20%, but one may be
making assessments that can be confirmed by independent assessment, while the other may be making almost random assessments.

In the research that I have carried out over the past
decade , I have used a self-administered psychiatric screening
questionnaire as an independent measure of psychiatric morbidity. The form which has been used most widely in this country
is the GHQ-60, which takes about 12 minutes to complete and
has been shown to have high reliability and validity. It was
especially designed for use in the general practitioner's
surgery, and has an unusual form of response scale. Most such
questionnaires use either frequency scales (ranging from "not
at all" to "continuously") or intensity scales (from "not at
all" to "extremely") in order to rate each symptom. The GHQ,
on the other hand, asks the respondent to compare his present
state to his usual state. Symptoms are only counted if the
patient is experiencing them "more than usual" or "much more
than usual".

The disadvantage of this form of scale is that patients
with acute disorders which may be about to resolve spontane-
ously will none the less be declared "cases" (and thus be
false positives) while those who have had symptoms for so many
years that they regard them as their "usual self" will be
declared non-cases (and thus be false negatives). However, it
may be of interest to study the former, and the family doctor
will always be aware of the identities of the latter! Against
these disadvantages there is a very real advantage. In the
setting of general practice, the GHQ works better. In one
study in which both the GHQ and a shortened version of the
SCL-90 were compared as possible screening tests, it was found
that there were fewer false positives with the GHQ.

The GHQ can be used to measure the *accuracy* of a doctor's
ratings of psychiatric disturbance among his patients. If the
doctor is asked to make a rating on a 6 point scale of the
degree of psychiatric disturbance of each patient he sees,
then these ratings can be compared with the patients' scores
on the GHQ. It is known that scores on the GHQ correlate
highly with blind, independent assessments made by research
psychiatrists using structured research interviews such as

the PSE or the CIS. Agreement between doctor and questionnaire
can be measured by correlation coefficients, which take a value
of zero if there is no association between two variables, and
unity if there is complete correspondence.

In our study of 91 general practitioners in Greater Manchester, we were able to show that some doctors had correlation
coefficients as high as psychistrists with unlimited time and
using research interviews, while others had a very poor relationship between their assessments and their patients' symptoms
Figure 1 shows the correlation coefficient obtained by these
doctors, with the coefficients of 45 American family practice
residents shown for comparison.

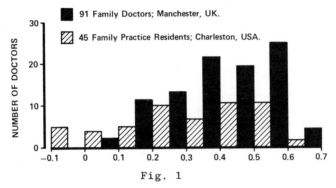

Fig. 1

The mean correlation coefficient for the Manchester doctors
is +0.39. There is a wide range - from +0.09 to +0.66 - and
the standard deviation is 0.15. We were able to account for
two-thirds of the variation between doctors in terms of 2
groups of factors - one concerning the way in which a doctor
interviewed his patients, and the other related to his personality.

Doctors who were rated by an independent observer as
"empathic", who asked about the patient's home and family, and
who tended to ask questions which related to the patient's
psychological adjustment, were better able to make accurate
assessments of emotional ill health. The personality variable
which turned out to be important was "conservatism", which is
not a measure of voting habits, but is conceived as a broad
personality dimension which reflects inflexibility, resistance
to change, and authoritarianism. Conservative doctors are
less likely to ask questions with a psychiatric content, and
make less accurate ratings of emotional illness.

This study has been repeated with family practice residents
in training at Charleston, South Carolina. On this occasion
we were able to use a rather more comprehensive set of personality tests for the doctor, and found that self-confident

doctors, who were able to handle their own feelings, were more
likely to make accurate assessments. Once more, doctors with
certain abilities as an interviewer were also more accurate.
These behaviours included making eye contact with the patient
at outset, using directive rather than closed questions,
tending to delay closed questions until they had given the
patient an opportunity to say what was on his mind by using
directive questions, and making sure that they clarified the
patient's complaint at the beginning of the interview. Such
doctors tended not to bury themselves in the notes while the
patient was talking, were able to handle garrulous patients,
and dealt with interruptions to their interview well. Finally,
they had a good knowledge of general medicine and a fairly
accurate concept of the kind of symptoms which characterize
psychiatric illness in this setting.

The final stage of the Charleston research was an intervention study. We identified the 24 doctors who were least able
to make accurate assessments of disorder from the entire set
of 45 doctors. We then randomly assigned the doctors to an
index training where they received special training sessions
from myself, and a control condition where they attended the
usual teaching programme but had no special sessions. The
special teaching was derived from work we have carried out
with undergraduates in Manchester, and makes extensive use of
video-taped feedback of their interview behaviour.

Each doctor received 4 teaching sessions. In the first
they were presented with a simple model for making psychiatric
assessments in a general practice setting, and were told the
desirable behaviours which I hoped to teach them. They were
shown video tapes of themselves which had been edited by myself so that they saw several behaviours which I wanted them
to lose. I should perhaps say that it took me several hours
to find suitable excerpts to show each doctor, taken from 5
different diagnostic interviews which had been seen by the
research team. Typical "bad" behaviours were starting the
interview with closed questions (e.g. "How are those headaches
of yours getting on?"; "Are you managing to stick to that
diet I gave you last time?"); failing to clarify the exact
nature of the patient's presenting complaint; failing to probe
verbal cues relating to psychiatric illness; failing to notice
gross non-verbal cues suggesting anxiety or depression; allowing the patient to go on giving the history while the doctor
reads the notes, and allowing over-talkative patients to
introduce irrelevant material which could not possibly help
them to reach a useful conclusion.

As you might guess, this first session could easily be
traumatic. For this reason I went out of my way also to show
them things that they did well, and tried to be fairly specific

about the behaviours that each doctor needed to learn. Over
the next three weeks, I made further recordings of their interviews, and once more, selected excerpts to show them during
sessions with me. If some behaviours seemed to cause difficulty, I would role play the patient myself and get them to
practise the particular behaviour. This device is known as
"microteaching", and is quite effective for the majority of
the students. However, some doctors were self-conscious and
in these cases I did not insist. After the 4 sessions - a
total of about 3 hours tuition - we reassessed the abilities
of the entire group of 24 doctors in terms of the accuracy of
their assessments of a new set of patients. The control group
were if anything worse, but the index group were much better.
The teaching had been a success.

However, it is worth recording that the effectiveness of
the teaching was because 5 of the 12 doctors in the index
groups had become very much more accurate in making assessments.
We tested the hypothesis that the doctors who had been best at
learning new interview behaviours were those who became most
accurate in making assessments: but this turned out not to be
the case. All the doctors had learned new techniques, but
only some of them had made use of their new insights, and conceptualized their patients in a new way. We could not tell
whether additional sessions would have helped the 7 index
doctors who did not become more accurate, nor could we tell
whether the beneficial effects of the teaching would be long
lasting.

Nevertheless, it is possible to give a list of 10 behaviours
which are not only highly related to a doctor's ability to
make accurate diagnostic assessments, but which can be modified
by a short course of training sessions. These are shown in
Table 1.

This table calls for some explanation. First, what suggested such behaviours to us in the first place? The answer
to this is that they arose from an earlier study of experienced
general practitioners in Manchester, and partly from our
research with medical students. There are more than 10
behaviours which relate to accuracy, but these are the only
ones that we were able to modify during training.

The idea of an "open-to-closed cone" derives from our work
with medical interviewing, and relates to the sequence of a
doctor's questions. The doctor should begin with open questions, and when he has heard the general nature of the presenting complaint should follow with directive questions. A
"directive" question indicates the aspect of the patient's
complaint which interests the doctor, but it unlike a "closed"
question since it cannot be answered with a simple "yes" or
"no". For example, "Describe the pain in your left arm" would

TABLE 1

Ten medical behaviours which relate to accuracy of
psychological assessment and which can be
significantly improved by training

Start of the interview:

1. Making eye contact with the patient

2. Clarification of the presenting complaint

Form of the "problem solving" questions:

3. Proportion directive (rather than closed)

4. Use of directive questions when dealing with
    physical symptoms

5. "Open to closed cones" (see text)

6. Focussing on the present rather than the past

Some special techniques

7. Sensitivity to verbal cues relating to psychological
    distress

8. Sensitivity to non-verbal cues indicating distress

9. Ability to deal with over-talkative patients

10. Ability to handle the notes (see text)

---

be directive; while "Was the pain in your left arm sharp or
dull?" would be closed. Doctors who are not very good at
making psychological assessments ask many closed questions,
and tend to ask them quite early in a sequence of questions –
without giving the patient an opportunity to express himself
in his own words.

"Focussing on the present" was measured by counting the
number of "past medical history" questions asked in the first
10 minutes of a diagnostic interview. Doctors who were not
good at making accurate assessments asked an astonishing
average of 33 such questions, but after training this had
dropped to a more moderate 13!

Over-talkative patients caused problems for inexperienced
interviewers, who sat transfixed before them, like rabbits
confronted with a cobra. It was fairly easy to teach them to
wait for a pause in the patient's speech, and to come in with
a directive question asked in a firm, polite manner. We also

observed that less able doctors tended to bury themselves in the notes while the patient was giving the history. They thought that they were listening to what the patient was saying, but of course they were not. Once more, it was a simple matter to teach them to ask the patient to pause while they looked up something in his notes.

The results of this study suggest that it would be desirable for family doctors in training to be given systematic instructions on their interview techniques. Theoretical lectures are quite useless for this purpose. To be effective, teaching must be directed at the point of delivery of service. In practice, this means audiotaped or video-taped recordings made of actual interviews with patients, which can then be discussed with a teacher in a small supervision group.

FURTHER READING

A comprehensive account of this research, with a complete review of the relevant literature, is to be found in "Mental Illness in the Community" by D. Goldberg and P. Huxley; published by Tavistock in 1980.

PSYCHIATRIC ILLNESS IN GENERAL PRACTICE

John Fry

138 Croydon Road,
Beckenham, Kent BR3 4DG

When first I started in my general practice over 30 years ago
I experienced a profound shock reaction because of the mass
of unfamiliar and unexpected conditions and situations that I
encountered.

Nowhere was my confusion and uncertainty greater than with
psycho-emotional-social problems. The features causing particular difficulties were:

1. their unexpectedly high prevalence;
2. their unfamiliar presentation;
3. their uncertain course and outcome;
4. problems of satisfactory management and care;
5. confusion over classification and nomenclature.

Many of these difficulties are still there but I would like
to share with you my current views based on more than 30 years
of study into these and other conditions in my practice over
this period.

WHAT IS GENERAL PRACTICE?

General practice, or primary care, is a special field of health
care that is essential in every health care system whatever
its political, social or economic organization-administration.

In every system there has to be someone to act as the primary health care worker who sees the patient in the first
instance, who is available and accessible, who works with a
relatively small and static population base, who provides
continuity of care and who is able to deal with the more
common and less dramatic diseases and disorders in the community and protect the more expensive hospital-specialist services
from inappropriate and wasteful work.

In Britain we have general practice that has evolved over
many generations to provide such primary care and in the

National Health Service (NHS) the general practitioner provides the greatest proportion of care for persons with psycho-
emotional illnesses. In the NHS there are particular opportunities to offer first contact care, to provide long term
and continuing care to a small and stable population and to
study and record the nature, course and outcome of such illnesses.

SOME FACTS AND MISFACTS

The following is a brief summary of psycho-emotional illness
as seen in general practice:

1. there are now approximately 2250 persons per GP in the NHS;
2. the prevalence of "labelled" overt psycho-emotional illness
   in general practice is probably between 100-150 per 1000
   and this means that one GP will meet and manage about 300
   persons each year with such conditions. Each may require
   a number of consultations;
3. contrary to some expectations there has been no increase
   in prevalence of psychiatric disorder diagnosis in my
   practice over 30 years - it has remained steady at around
   10% of all consultations in any and every year;
4. in addition there are likely to be as many if not more
   persons with psycho-emotional problems who attend for
   various systems and whose true nature is unrecognized;
5. further, there must be more persons in the community with
   these conditions who do not seek help or advice;
6. only about 1 in 20 (5%) of these persons are referred to
   a psychiatrist in any year. The GP manages 95% without
   referral;
7. drug therapy has changed remarkably in content but less
   remarkably in volume. Thirty years ago the common psychotropics used in general practice were barbiturates and
   bromides and they appeared to help patients and doctors.
   Now both groups have been all but abandoned and replaced
   by wide ranges of tranquillizing and antidepressant drugs.
   In total volume of prescriptions for psychotropic drugs
   in the NHS by general practitioners there has been no
   great change. We appear to prescribe as many modern psychotropics now as we did barbiturates and bromides in the
   1950s.

WHAT IS GENERAL PRACTICE PSYCHIATRY?

A major problem with psychiatry in general and with general
practice psychiatry in particular is that the conditions and
situations encountered exist as descriptive collections largely

of symptoms and a few signs with little correlation with any
substantive pathological or biochemical changes. It is not
possible to be precise in definitive diagnosis or apply good
objective measures for degrees of severity.

The nomenclature and classifications that we are offered
exemplify these problems - anxiety, depression, obsessions,
phobias, grief, bereavement, personality disorders and others.

Psychiatry in general practice broadly deals with vulnerable individuals and families who present problems, difficulties and reactions from stresses and strains within their
personal environments. They may present with "anxiety",
"depression", "phobias", "obsessions" and "personality disorders" but they are individuals with problems that have to
be listened to, unravelled, and resolved (if possible) with
assistance. They are families and individuals that have to
be supported and accepted over many, many years.

But in spite of such unhelpful nomenclature there are certain guidelines that emerge from long term observations in
general practice.

The *age-prevalance* of psycho-emotional problems is that
although they occur at all ages the peak-prevalence is between
the 25 and 55 year period.

There is a very definite *sex predominance* of females by as
much as 3:1 - particularly at the peak 25-55 age-group.

The *natural course* and *outcome* tend to follow a rule of
3 thirds:

1. about one-third of persons with psycho-emotional illnesses
   in general practice will experience a *single appreciable
   attack* and then never again suffer;
2. about one-third will suffer *recurring episodes* of depres-
   sion-anxiety over many years;
3. about one-third will become *chronic* and have continual
   symptoms and problems over many, many years.

The *management* of these persons in uncertain, unclear and
unproven. Each general practitioner develops his own approach
related to his own personality, philosophy and understanding
of these conditions.

The essences are:

1. psychotherapy and support;
2. use of psychotropic drugs;
3. enlistment of help from other agencies and persons.

The *results of care* also are uncertain, unclear and unproven,
and it is impossible to apportion credits to any specific form
of therapy.

CURRENT PROBLEMS AND ISSUES

My contribution intentionally seeks to raise issues and problems that require planned support and research to resolve them and to assist us all in better care, management and prevention of psycho-emotional illnesses in our community, based on sound sense and sensibility.

I shall list these and add some comments:

1. *What are psychiatric illnesses?*
   We cannot assume that because the ICD (International Classification of Diseases) has a large category for these conditions that we know to what they refer and that we know their pathogenesis and their true nature. Much more study and effort are required to add to knowledge and understanding and much of this work must be carried out in general practice where 95% of the conditions are managed.

2. *What is their natural history?*
   If we are to be able to manage psychiatric illnesses effectively, efficiently and economically we need better baselines of their natural history, without the effects of specific therapies. We must know whether our therapies are any improvement on natural history. Once again such studies can only be carried out in general practice in collaboration with academic units.

3. *Who should carry out what care where, when, how and why?*
   It would be wrong to assume that only GPs or psychiatrists can manage successfully such illnesses. There are many others in the medico-social spectrum who may be better or equal in providing care - such as nurses, social workers, clinical psychologists, counsellors and members of the many and various fringe medicine cults. Trials and experiments should be conducted to assess how care can be shared or delegated for optimal results.

4. *What is useful and what is useless?*
   As specific extension of trials and experiments we must be prepared to be much more critical in a constructive manner, of present (and future) trends in care. Some have little objective evidence of any real benefit and should be scrapped.

5. *Whose responsibilities?*
   In sharing and allocating care it is important to apportion responsibilities not only between professional groups but also to make sure that the individual realizes his/her own responsibilities for health attainment, health maintenance, disease prevention and co-operation with professional groups.

WHAT ROLES AND ACTIONS FOR THE MHF?

To begin to undertake some of these studies; to try to answer such questions needs action, stimulus and support of some grant-giving body such as the MHF.

Not everything can or should be supported because funds are limited, but planned policies should be developed to stimulate research in this field.

I hope that the wise move to hold this conference will provide the stimulus to create plans and priorities for support of research into psychiatric disorders in the community in general and in general practice in particular. My hope extends beyond the limit of the MHF. The MHF should take the lead and now go ahead and prepare guidelines for such research and then call together another small conference of all grant supporting bodies interested in the field and stimulate them into the joint actions required to study the problems referred to and to produce actions for better care.

SESSION I
GENERAL DISCUSSION

Dr Barbara BURNS (National Institute of Mental Health, USA):
Since my discussion comes from an American perspective, may I
quote from a 1920 novel by Sinclair Lewis on the role of the
GP:

> Great work these country practitioners are doing. The
> other day in Washington I was talking to a big scien-
> tific shot at Johns Hopkins Medical School. He was say-
> ing that no one had ever sufficiently appreciated the
> general practitioner and the sympathy and help he gives
> folks. These crack specialists, the young scientific
> fellows, are so cock-sure and so wrapped up in their
> laboratories that they miss the human element, except
> in the case of a few freak diseases that no one in
> their rightful mind would consider wasting his time
> having. It is the old "doc" who keeps the community
> well, mind and body.

The challenge in 1981 is to maximize that human element while
also incorporating new knowledge from epidemiology, from
behavioural sciences and from psychiatry. A difficult question facing general practice is whether the art of the doctor/
patient relationship can truly benefit from the science of
those fields even though that science may sometimes, as we
heard this morning, be somewhat undeveloped. However, if we
can definitely address some of the questions raised we should
make important headway in the improved detection, diagnosis
and management of emotional problems and mental disorder in
general practice patients.
 The problems that were addressed this morning were three-
fold: the nature and extent of mental disorders in general
practice; naming those disorders; dealing with them.
 With respect to extent and nature, it was reassuring to
hear Dr Fry say that the prevalence has been unchanged for
30 years. One statistic claimed is that psychiatric problems
comprise 50% of consultations. The situation becomes
frightening as the general practitioner and the mental health

professionals are both in danger of being overwhelmed clinically. We must heed reports such as the recent Primary Care
Survey in London which concluded that mental disorder was
twice as common in London as in outer areas. But the issue
is not the extent but the nature of the disorder.

Dr Ingham impressed on us the need to differentiate the
ill from the non-ill. We cannot afford management efforts
when they are likely to be ineffective. There are 3 groups
of patients: those with a true psychiatric disorder; those
with medical problems; and those with medical problems with
psychological factors, life problems and crises. Major attention should be given to the minor disorders in general practice. We conducted a study several years ago using the SADS,
mentioned by Dr Ingham, administered to people in a large pre-
paid health plan, and found an annual prevalence of 27%. Nine
percent had major affective disorders, 9% minor depressive
disorders, and the remaining 9% comprised anxiety, phobia and
other disorders.

The second question concerned nomenclature. Dr Clare
claimed we are missing serious disorders. The WHO project
that he talked about aims to classify mental disorders by
starting at the symptom level, but allowing the diagnostic
process to allow for changes over time.

Another point of Dr Clare's I disagree with - whether
anxiety-depressions seen in primary care are different from
those conditions seen in psychiatric populations. That is an
empirical question, and, as the data I have just cited show,
high rates of the more serious disorders are found in primary
care.

The third question raised by Professor Goldberg and Dr Fry
was what to do. Professor Goldberg demonstrated that through
special training in interview skills detection can be improved.
In earlier work with Dr Goldstone, he provided simple feed-
back from the General Health Questionnaire and thereby improved
detection and treatment. The issues of detection and treatment, however, have been less thoroughly addressed through
control studies. The critical issue concerning the practitioner is the relevance of the epidemiological work to clinical
practice. Professor Goldberg's work has demonstrated the
principle. There may be ways to incorporate such work into
conceptual models for the clinician which begin to relate
emotional and psychiatric problems to the necessary therapeutic
approaches.

Finally, a practical thing needs to be kept in mind, to
sort out what is already known with clear immediate clinical
implications from the research agenda provided for us by Dr
Fry and by the other 3 lecturers this morning.

Dr Godfrey FOWLER (Oxford): Was any form of patient assessment of interviews introduced into Professor Goldberg's interview training; secondly has he any evidence that the training
improved patient satisfaction with the interview?

Professor Goldberg: The training was entirely based on patient
interview but we do not know what effect training had on
patient satisfaction.

Dr Thomas PASTOR (London): I have a session in general practice where I see patients, much as I do in psychiatric out-
patient clinics. My concern is to identify problems which can
be treated effectively by the general practitioner and also to
advise on referral to other resources, particularly for psychotherapy. I am increasingly anxious at the way that the problem of psychiatric illness in general practice is diffusing
outwards. For example, we are told to bring social factors
into the way we classify problems in general practice. But
what do we do when we define it in that way? Psychiatric
illness slips out of our hands and becomes a problem for
social workers, not for doctors. Part of the problem may be
that we need to define how we define illness. In psychiatry
we define it by recognizing a symptom. But in a way, illness
is often defined not in medical terms but in social terms.
The way we say somebody is ill is by the way they behave; they
show illness behaviour.

Dr Brendan KELLY (Merthyr Tydfil): I see mental illness in
practice in 2 ways. The psychoses are dealt with very effectively because they are diagnosed by a consultant psychiatrist
and the only object is to keep them on treatment and prevent
further breakdowns. But neurosis in general practice is a
much more difficult problem, mainly because it is often not
regarded by the patient as a legitimate illness to come with
to the doctor.

Dr Anthony CLIFT (Manchester): Dr Fry raised an interesting
point, namely that the prevalence of psycho-emotional conditions has not changed over some years. That is our experience
too from the data in our morbidity register. Can the same be
said for the situation in the community? There is a sort of
tolerance to psycho-emotional conditions that GPs will cope
with, but when the prevalence exceeds about 20% GPs change to
an organic diagnosis.

Dr Fry: The expectations of the public are something that we
do not fully appreciate. It has become more respectable for
the public to suffer from emotional illnesses due to the
influence of the media.

Professor GOLDBERG: Dr Clift remarked that after a certain point a GP cuts out and makes organic diagnoses. This cut-out reaction is a serious phenomenon in doctors who do not know what to do about emotional disorder and feel threatened by it. Now regarding what Tony Clare said about tri-axial diagnosis, sooner or later the general practitioner will say "What difference does tri-axial diagnosis make to patient care? Unless epidemiologists tell general practitioners what tri-axial diagnosis will mean in terms of management skills, it will be a worthless research tool.

Dr Fry said that what matters is the way young doctors are paid. Now I have watched overworked colleagues in Greater Manchester under the National Health Service, and I have watched exceedingly well paid and leisured colleagues in the United States. My conclusions obtained in both countries, irrespective of the way the doctors were being paid. However, the way a doctor is paid makes a great difference to the quality of service.

Mrs Elizabeth MITCHELL (London): The medical model is still used in epidemiological studies in assuming that mental illness will eventually carry with it some prospects of cure. The notion of cure was raised earlier in the discussion and is important in devising appropriate criteria of change, educating the patient, and in eliminating inappropriate expectations. But in terms of treatment the crisis intervention, for example, works from a totally different perspective, looking not at long-term criteria of change but at the short-term.

Dr June HUNTINGTON (Sydney, Australia): In Australia at the moment there is a doctor/patient ratio of 1 to under 1400. The GPs there say that Australia is becoming over-doctored. Some parts of the profession respond by moving into the counselling area, helped by the tripartite fee structure that Dr Fry mentioned. Now there are people who need the counselling but the GPs will concentrate on the psychological side and neglect the social side. They will remain on a one-to-one clinical level but will not look at the social environment in which the patient or client currently lives.

SESSION II

MANAGEMENT OF PSYCHIATRIC ILLNESS IN GENERAL PRACTICE

Luke Zander

*Department of General Practice,
St Thomas's Hospital Medical School,
80 Kennington Road, London SE11 4TH*

The study of the epidemiology of psychiatric illness is fraught with problems of definition and classification. The relevance of this to the practising physician is that diagnosis is the precursor to treatment and the way in which a particular presenting symptom or symptom complex is perceived will in large part determine the type of management prescribed. Some of the differences and difficulties that have been identified represent fundamental problems when considering the management of psychiatric illness or psychological disorders presenting in the setting of general practice.

In considering the treatment that is available, I would like to do more than purely consider the options open to the primary health care team and would like to rephrase the title in the form of a question, "How would we, as a multi-disciplinary group, approach the task of improving the management of psychological problems, or even more positively, improving the level of mental health in the community for which we are responsible?" As in so many other aspects of medical care, it is not the lack of knowledge which is so often the determining factor in what we do, but the problems and difficulties related to the process of care. Therefore, it is of extreme importance that we identify and grapple with some of the real difficulties that faces one in attempting to provide the optimal type of care.

MANAGEMENT IN THE CONSULTING ROOM

It is well known that overt psychological problems and stress related disorders represent a major component of the symptoms presenting to the general practitioner (Shepherd *et al.*, 1966;

Morrell *et al.*, 1971). Also, when considering the factors
which influence the demand for medical care, anxiety has been
shown to be very significant (Banks *et al.*, 1975).

What options are open to the practitioner if he wishes to
undertake the care of his patient himself? He can either
give a prescription or undertake some form of psychotherapy
(using this term in its widest form). The question of prescribing is being considered in detail by Professor Parish,
but I would just like to make an observation from the perspective of the practitioner. There are very few doctors who are
unaware of the problems associated with the prescribing of
tranquillizers and antidepressants, and who would not give
very adequate answers, if posed theoretical questions about
their usage. However, we need to understand that the pressure
to prescribe a tranquillizer is almost as great as the com-
pulsion the patient has to going on taking it. If it is felt
appropriate to provide some form of prescription, we need to
consider how to avoid the possibility of this becoming a start
to the repeat prescription merry-go-round.

Varnam (1981) described a process of audit that he has
undertaken as the initial step in modifying his prescribing
habits. Harris at St Mary's Hospital undertook a project
involving 50 general practitioners in discussions about their
prescribing habits together with feed-back information about
their prescriptions. He found that their prescribing was
markedly altered. The increasing interest in audit, particularly if it is of an educational rather than a punitive nature,
could provide an important stimulus for improvement in our
prescribing.

Whether or not we believe in the views of Illich and others
about the dangers of the medicalization of the problems of
life, the reality is that we are often confronted by them and
therefore, the appropriate question is not should we be dealing with them, but how can we provide the appropriate care.
I would like to consider briefly the educational model and
pose the question, "What is the sort of educational programme
that we should devise with this objective in mind?" We have
now established a 3 year compulsory vocational training programme, one year of which is spent in practice and 2 years in
rotating hospital posts. In many schemes in the country,
psychiatry is one of the options of these 2 years and the
Royal Colleges of Psychiatrists and General Practitioners
have together produced a document, outlining the experience
that they feel is desirable for the general practice trainee
occupying a SHO post (Working Party, 1978). They state that
during a 6 month appointment is should be possible to obtain
worthwhile experience in the following areas:

1. General Psychiatric Practice, including interview techniques, taking case histories and making formal diagnosis;
2. Methods of Psychiatric Treatment, especially the proper
   use of psychotropic medication and of the more simple
   psychotherapeutic procedures.

It is, however, recognized that "the trainee cannot hope
to obtain sufficient counselling expertise within such
appointments".

What is the result of such a 6 month attachment? My own
feeling is that it can be counter-productive because although
the knowledge of the trainee is increased, his attitude and
perception about psychological disorders is frequently modified in a direction inappropriate to the general practice
setting. All too frequently, the emphasis is on making a
diagnosis in disease or pathological terms, such as depression
or anxiety, rather than on a careful assessment and examination of the possible aetiological factors. It is this which
so often leads them understandably to adopt an almost reflex
reaction to prescribe something to relieve the symptom. In
making this statement I am not arguing for doing away with
the psychiatric input into the vocational training programme,
but am suggesting that we need to consider very carefully
what its contents should be, and if it is felt that the hospital setting is an inappropriate one in which to develop
certain attitudes or skills, then we need to identify how and
where these can better be learned. It was interesting to
find during a year working in London, Ontario, that the Resi-
dency or Trainee programme had no formal attachment to a
psychiatric unit, but very considerable effort was made
throughout the 2 years to develop the doctor's ability in
communication and counselling skills. Because of the setting
of this conference, it is appropriate to mention in this context that the Oxford region is giving a lead to the rest of
the country in developing ways by which the interviewing and
consulting skills of trainees can be improved by sophisticated
teaching programmes involving the use of video recordings of
consultations, and this is now part of the vocational training programme throughout the region.

AVAILABILITY OF TIME

One of the reasons most commonly given for being unable to
undertake certain activities or procedures in general practice is the lack of time. It is true that this is an
exceedingly valuable commodity, but one is less convinced
that the way in which it is used is given the consideration
that it deserves. The utilization of time is a question

which deserves much thought. Since having trainees I have asked myself what is it in fact that one does which couldn't be done just as well or even better by others? While it is probably fair to say that a large number of consultations could be equally well undertaken by the trainee, an experienced doctor or even the practice nurse, there are certain things which could probably be done better by a trainee who has just completed his hospital training, and there are others for which the experienced practitioner is likely to be better equipped. I suggest that these lie in the areas of understanding human behaviour, which comes from having spent many years responsible for the care of individuals experiencing illness, disease, birth, death and other of life's major events. Hopefully, over time one increases one's sensitivity and understanding of inter-personal relationships and psychodynamics. If that is so, it is surely important that we should ensure that more of our time is taken up in this type of activity. This has certain implications, as it means that we can no longer take a completely passive role in deciding how our time is to be used. At present most doctors take little part in organizing the distribution of their consultation time, but leave it to the patients to make whatever demands they feel appropriate. If one is really to maximize one's effectiveness in the areas of psychotherapy a change of approach is necessary. This is not to suggest that there should be a filter mechanism which directs patients to different providers of care on a basis of hierarchy of experience, but rather that one puts certain periods of time aside to undertake particular forms of activity. Most doctors will occasionally get patients back for a long consultation, by having, for instance, one session a week for such consultations, as at present, one puts time aside for ante-natal or well baby clinics. It is likely that if this was part of the timetable, one's willingness to undertake this form of care would be much increased.

THE INTER-RELATIONSHIP BETWEEN GENERAL PRACTITIONER AND SPECIALIST SERVICES

The nature of interaction between the primary and secondary levels of care is relevant to all aspects of medicine but perhaps, particularly to those branches such as mental health, where the respective roles of each are so much less clearly delineated. As was stated in a WHO document in 1973 (WHO, 1973):

> The primary care team is the keystone in community psychiatry; the crucial question is not how the general practitioner can fit into the mental health services,

but rather how the psychiatrist can collaborate most
effectively with primary medical care.

Professor Cooper, elsewhere in this book, considers the question of referral to psychiatric services from general practice
but there is one specific aspect that I would like to focus
attention on. It is inevitable that the vast majority of
psychological problems will have to and can most appropriately
be dealt with in primary care and it is significant, therefore,
to consider to what extent the specialist services can themselves contribute to improving the capability of the primary
physician.

In the normal situation when a practitioner asks the help
and advice of his specialist colleagues, he must refer
the patient to the hospital setting with the obvious
associated disadvantages, e.g. lack of communication between
the clinicians concerned, delay before the patient is seen,
the number of different personnel that my be involved in the
patient's continuing care and the possible stigma associated
with the referral. A number of experiments for reducing these
problems have been undertaken. In Edinburgh, psychiatric
teams have been responsible for individual sectors of the
town, thereby improving the relationship and communication
between the local practitioners and the members of a psychiatric team. At St Thomas's an experiment of giving general
practitioners direct access to a consultant emergency psychiatric clinic was established in order to reduce the problem
of delay. A different approach involves the specialist services coming out into the community. This is the principle
which lay behind the concept of the Health Centre, the belief
that if the specialist and primary care services are undertaken in the same setting, many of the above problems would
be reduced.

However, a more sophisticated and fundamentally different
approach to the problem was developed by Dr Alexis Brook
(Brook and Temperley, 1976) of the Community Adult Unit of
the Taverstock Clinic, in the early 70s, in which he undertook to provide psychiatric support for general practitioners,
in the setting of their own practices. The importance of
this lay in the fact that they were attending not as specialists providing specialist care for the patients, but as consultants to the general practitioner. The consultant would
see any patient referred to him for one or 2 assessment interviews only, following which he and the general practitioner
would discuss together the appropriate alternative forms of
management. The patient would then only be seen again by the
psychiatrist if the general practitioner felt this would be
helpful to review progress. Besides the obvious advantages of

accessibility, shorter waiting times, and reduced chance of seeing different psychiatrists, the main benefit to be derived
from this arrangement was that there was a sharing of knowledge
between the 2 clinicians and the development of a mutual educa-
tive process, by which the general practitioner was encouraged
and helped to develop further his competence and confidence in
providing the care for his patients. This is a model of care
that has general applicability and the Department of General
Practice at St Thomas's has developed similar schemes for the
management of diabetes, ante-natal care and the monitoring of
the care of epileptics. It is an arrangement that has been
shown to be logistically feasible, and deserves most serious
consideration.

THE USE OF THE PRIMARY HEALTH CARE TEAM

The underlying principle of the primary health care team is
that there are different aspects of medical care that can most
appropriately be undertaken by individuals with different
skills and perspectives, and that by working together in close
proximity, the overall care of the patient is enhanced. This
concept has now become generally accepted, with the rapid
development of Group Practices and the attachment of para-
medical staff, principally health visitors, nurses and to a
lesser extent, midwives and social workers.

An interesting development in the field of management of
psychological problems has been the more recent experience
with the attachment of psychologists and counsellors. The
involvement of counsellors is considered elsewhere in this
book by Dr Pamela Ashurst and I would only like to make some
very general comments from the standpoint of the practitioner.
The results of introducing individuals with these specific
skills has been shown to be successful (Trethowan, 1977), as
judged by a reduction in the prescribing of psychotropic medication and in the fall in the consultation rates to the practitioner (Johnstone, 1978).

However, one must be aware of the possible reaction against
this type of attachment if one is to hope for its more general
application. At a recent meeting at The Royal Society of
Medicine, where the benefits to be derived from the introduction of individuals with such skills was discussed by Dr John
Hasler and a Counsellor, Sally Ann Anderson, who had attempted
to evaluate such an attachment (Hasler and Anderson, 1979),
there was very definite opposition to their introduction into
the health care team. This was based on the belief that if
we proceed along this line the very *raison d'être* of the
generalist would be threatened. This response represents a
misunderstanding of the potential benefit of such an arrange-

ment in that it is not suggested that a particular range of problems would automatically be referred to or dealt with by the psychologists or counsellor, but rather that they would be available as a resource to patient or practitioners if and when required. An interesting, but not unexpected, finding was that in fact the generalists undertook more care of behavioural problems following the attachment of a counsellor than beforehand, indicating that her presence had increased the doctor's sensitivity and confidence in dealing with such problems. After the experimental period was over, there was an unanimous feeling that the attachment should be continued.

Involvement of clinical psychologists into primary care is a comparatively new development, but one which would seem to have very real potential. Marie Johnstone (1978) of the Department of Psychiatry at The Royal Free Hospital, included among the advantages of such an attachment:

1. access to psychological help for patients who could not attend the central clinic, owing to problems associated with travel, work, physical disability or even a presenting problem, such as agrophobia;
2. increased communication between the psychologists and members of the primary health care team;
3. possibility of the psychologist seeing the patient earlier, before the problems become too entrenched;
4. reduced stigma for the patient;
5. development of new therapeutic approaches relevant to problems presenting in primary care;
6. more flexible and more relevant therapy due to seeing patients in their home setting.

The Trethowan Committee (Trethowan, 1977), reporting about the work of clinical psychologists, recommended that they should work more closely with general practitioners. In addition to general counselling skills, clinical psychologists are equipped with rapid treatment methods which are effective in the common neurotic disorders. In his study in Sheffield, Koch noted that a reduction in consultations to the doctor and prescriptions dispensed were maintained a year later (Koch, 1979). He estimated that 10 to 15 clinical psychologists would be adequate for a city of that size. At present the financing of such an attachment is not covered by the normal NHS reimbursement scheme, but it is an issue that could with great benefit be the subject of central discussion. It would seem that such a development would have the support of clinical psychologists because in this setting they would assume less of a secondary role than they may have to adopt in a psychiatric hospital. The problem of increasing their utilization might well lie in opposition from the general practitioners (as in the case of counsellors). This may in part be based on ignorance and would indicate a need for some early exposure to the potential role of psychologists, ideally during the vocational training period.

ALTERNATIVE APPROACHES TO MEDICAL CARE

It is now hardly possible to pick up a medical or lay journal without finding some reference to alternative medicine. It is an issue which touches on many fundamental questions relating not just to therapeutics or the management of disease, but to the basic principles which underlie our concepts of illness and how the profession should respond to unorthodox approaches to care. It is interesting to note that there are now as many practitioners of unorthodox medicine as there are GPs, and whatever we ourselves feel about the therapeutic effectiveness or validity, of acupuncture, homeopathy, meditation, spiritualism, etc. they are forms of help that are increasingly being sought by our patients. Whereas up to a few years ago, there was little actual evidence to support them, there is now an increasing amount of scientific interest in trying to elucidate both whether and how they might work. Relaxation techniques, meditation, bio-feedback are all now the focus of much serious study. Dr Malcolm Carruthers, at the Maudsley, has shown the effects of behaviour modification, bio-feedback, autogenic training and meditation on levels of blood pressure, pulse rates, smoking habits, as well as on serum levels of cholesterol and free fatty acids. The cardiologist, Dr Peter Nixon, at Charing Cross Hospital, uses relaxation techniques as a major part of his post coronary therapy (Nixon, 1972), and Dr C. Patel, a general practitioner in South London, has shown striking effects of meditation in the treatment of hypertension (Patel and Carruthers, 1977). All these would seem to act by reducing levels of anxiety and stress. In our own practice, we undertook a small study, treating patients presenting with insomnia with relaxation instruction, and this produced a number of interesting findings:

1. nearly all patients showed a marked improvement in their sleeping habits;
2. patients were nearly all delighted not to have been prescribed hypnotics (although that is what many of them came requesting) when they were told that there was another type of treatment available for them;
3. many of them admitted using the relaxation techniques at other times of stress.

Is it possible to employ these techniques within a practice setting? Dr John English, a general practitioner in Middlesex, has a number of patient groups undertaking autogenic training for stress related disorders, and no doubt there are a number of others, such as Dr Patel. However, it would seem more likely that these are techniques that can well be undertaken outside the setting of the practice and as Dr Nixon has said, what we need is a pharmacopoeia of individuals with special interests and skills to whom we can refer our patients.

SUPPORT GROUPS

A very significant benefit can be derived from patients presenting with conditions such as depression, anxiety, bereavement, etc., by the support and encouragement derived from peer groups. The doctors may have no part to play in such a group, but may have a role in helping to initiate its establishment. Certain practices have established patient groups of this nature, but it is more likely that it will be the health visitor who has a particularly significant part to play in identifying such resources. In my own district of North Lambeth it has been very interesting to see the groups that have been established in response to a wide range of differing psychological needs and it is of extreme importance that we as practitioners are not only aware of the value of such groups, but show ourselves willing to become involved, if only in so far as to know of their existence and be prepared to direct our patients to them.

In summary, therefore, we need to consider how, as practitioners, we, or if not we, at least those coming after us, are to acquire the necessary skills to identify the nature of our patients' problems and then help in their resolution. How can we more effectively control our prescribing of psychotropic medication? How can we organize our primary and secondary levels of care, so that there is an economic use of resources and that each is able to function at their true potential? How can we develop the primary health care team so that we are more able to provide for our patients' psychological and behavioural problems, while still maintaining the essence of personal doctoring? In what way can we open our eyes to a wider horizon of therapeutic possibilities, whether in the form of new specific techniques or in a greater realization of the value to be gained from inter-personal support systems? It is through meetings of this nature, designed to stimulate inter-disciplinary discussion, that new ideas can be developed. I am sure that if these are to be put into practice, it is at the level of the new entrants to practice that we need to focus, and those of us concerned with education have a

responsibility to ensure that we do indeed try to train doctors
now entering our ranks to practise a type of medicine which
takes account of the contemporary and emerging ideas from a
wide front of human experience.

REFERENCES

Anderson, S. and Hasler, J.C. (1979). Counselling in general
  practice. *Journal of the Royal College of General Practitioners* **29**, 352-356.
Banks, M.H., Beresford, S.A., Morrell, D.C., Waller, J.J. and
  Watkins, C.J. (1975). Factors influencing demand for pri-
  mary medical care in women aged 20-44 years: a preliminary
  report. *International Journal of Epidemiology* **4** (3), 189-
  195.
Brook, A. and Temperley, J. (1976). The contribution of a
  psychotherapist to general practice. *Journal of the Royal
  College of General Practitioners* **26**, 86-94.
Harris, C.H. (1981). Personal communication.
Johnstone, M. (1978). The work of a clinical psychologist in
  primary care. *Journal of the Royal College of General
  Practitioners* **28**, 661-667.
Koch, H.C.H. (1979). Evaluation of behaviour therapy intervention in general practice. *Journal of the Royal College
  of General Practitioners* **29**, 337-340.
Morrell, D.C., Gage, H.G. and Robinson, N.A.A. (1971). Symp-
  toms in general practice. *Journal of the Royal College
  of General Practitioners* **21**, 32-43.
Nixon, P.G. (1972). Rehabilitation of the coronary patient.
  Physiotherapy **58**, 336-338.
Patel, C. and Carruthers, M. (1977). Coronary risk factor
  reduction through bio-feedback aided relaxation and medita-
  tion. *Journal of the Royal College of General Practitioners*
  27, 401-405.
Shepherd, M., Cooper, B., Brown, A.C. and Kalton, G.W. (1966).
  Psychiatric Illness in General Practice. Oxford University
  Press, London.
Trethowan, W.H. (1977). The role of the psychologist in the
  Health Service. HMSO, London.
Varnam, M. (1981). Psychotropic prescribing. What am I doing?
  Journal of the Royal College of General Practitioners **31**,
  480-483.
Working Party Report of RCGP and RCPSYCH. (1978). Training
  for general practitioner. Occasional Paper 6. *Journal of
  the Royal College of General Practitioners.*
World Health Organization (1973). Psychiatry and Primary
  Medical Care. WHO Regional Office for Europe, Copenhagen.

THE USE OF PSYCHOTROPIC DRUGS
IN GENERAL PRACTICE

Peter A. Parish

*Medicines Research Unit,
32 Park Place, Cardiff CF1 3BA*

Any discussion about the use of psychotropic drugs in general
practice usually becomes charged with emotion and results in
an inevitable process of polarization. Yet there is nothing
new about doctors using drugs to change the moods of their
patients nor is there anything new in patients taking mood
altering drugs. What is new is the sociological interest in
the use of these drugs and the identification of problems of
use often based on unsubstantiated evidence.

Certainly, a picture has emerged over the past 2 decades of
people experiencing a multitude of physical and mental symptoms for which they are offered relief in the form of psychotropic drugs (Parish, 1971; Dunnell and Cartwright, 1972;
Williams, 1978; Raynes, 1979; Anderson, 1980a). This has led
to concern about the amount of these drugs being prescribed
by general practitioners (Parish, 1971; Tomski, 1979; Williams,
1980). The intensity of market competition and sales promotion by drug companies have been blamed for this increase
(Parish, 1971), so too has the available number of different
drug preparations with similar effects (Tyrer, 1978). Doctors
also have been criticized for their generous and often indis-
criminate prescribing (Parish, 1971; Tyrer, 1978; Dennis,
1979).

Evidence of dependency to such drugs as the benzodiazepines
has been produced (Marks, 1978; Lader, 1980) and reports of
their increasing use in acts of self-poisoning has given rise
to concern (Hawton and Blackstock, 1977; Jones, 1977). It
has been shown that an increasing number of individuals take
psychotropic drugs regularly over many years (Parish, 1971;
Dunnell and Cartwright, 1972; Tyrer, 1978; Dennis, 1979;
Anderson, 1980b), and wastage in their use has been demonstrated by findings from unused drug collection programmes
(Wilson, 1972; Hughes, 1973) and studies cf patient non-com-
pliance (Blackwell, 1976; Haynes *et al.*, 1979).

The ease with which patients are able to obtain a repeat
supply has been highlighted (Austin and Parish, 1976; Freed,
1976; Dennis, 1979; Anderson, 1980b; Murdock, 1980), so too
has the observation that their consumption increases with the
advancing age of the individual (Parish, 1971; Skegg et al.,
1977) and that twice as many women as men take them (Parish,
1971; Skegg et al., 1977; Harris et al., 1977). Their use has
not been significantly correlated to any social variable and
despite a decade or more of prescribing studies we have made
little progress in really understanding the many factors which
influence the prescribing and use of these drugs.

We know that psychotropic drugs are being used increasingly
in many fields of contemporary therapeutics (Parish, 1971;
Skegg et al., 1977), that they are used more frequently than
any other group of drugs, and that patterns of their use in
most Western countries are similar (Wilcox, 1972; Parry et al.,
1973; Balter et al., 1974; Hemminki, 1974; Pflanz et al.,
1977; Webb, 1979; Grimsson et al., 1979). These patterns of
use suggest both distinctive trends in the type of psychotropic drug prescribed and a steady increase in their prescription (Parish, 1971; Williams, 1980).

In seeking to explain their increased use some observers
suggest that psychotropic drugs are being prescribed by
doctors instead of them taking time to counsel their patients
(Balint et al., 1970; Lader, 1978; Murdock, 1980) and it is
now frequently implied that it is easier to give a prescription than to give advice and that it is easier to take a pill
than take advice. This criticism is often aimed at the doctor
working in primary care in the British National Health Service
and yet in countries where private medicine operates and where
patients are given more time, the prescribing of these drugs
appears similar (Parry et al., 1973). It is also claimed
that because older doctors received no formal training in
learning to manage the burden of mental disorders and common
anxieties which exist in the community, they resort to phar-
macotherapy rather than psychotherapy (Balint et al., 1970;
Lader, 1978). Yet the prescribing of these drugs appears to
be no less amongst doctors with special interests in psychological disorders (Balint et al., 1970; Parish, 1971). The
suggestion that more time spent between doctor and patient
would result in a reduction in drug use remains to be proven.

However, by their use of these drugs, doctors clearly
define to patients a model for dealing with certain symptoms
produced by unpleasant situations. Doctors' prescribing
habits therefore influence patients' expectations which subsequently determine demands, although there is some evidence
of reduced expectations for drug treatments in recent years
(Cartwright and Anderson, 1981). Prescribing goes in fashions:

bromides, barbiturates, amphetamines, phenothiazines, MAOIs, tricyclics, benzodiazepines and tetracyclics. Along with changes in drug fashions, go changes in diagnostic labelling. These days doctors will seldom talk about neuraesthenia or nervous debility; they prefer to talk about anxiety and depression. But of course coping mechanisms may have changed as symptoms of stress have become defined and re-defined as requiring drug treatment. The threshold of tolerance of feelings may therefore have changed resulting in a greater demand for relief (Wadsworth *et al.*, 1970). Certainly, symptomatic treatment has increased, but in part this may be related to the availability of effective drugs. Furthermore, defined symptoms of emotional disorders are often insidious and run a protracted and episodic course. Many patients seek relief from such symptoms and present to their doctors regularly over time. Because of the availability of psychotropic drugs, these patients are treated with such drugs.

In addition to a possible change in the threshold of tolerance to feelings, the number of symptoms recognized as psychological has increased so that there is now hardly a physical or mental symptom which may not be regarded as psychological, indicating the need for psychotropic drug treatment. Drug companies have intensively and systematically taken everyday social situations and medical situations, particularly involving women, and indicated that such situations produce stress (Lennard *et al.*, 1971; Stimson, 1975; Cooperstock, 1978; King, 1980). At one and the same time, they have defined the victims of stress and the need to treat them with psychotropic drugs (Lennard *et al.*, 1971; Cooperstock and Lennard, 1979).

Against this background of created demand for the relief of symptoms of stress a fundamental question must be asked – how appropriate is it for doctors to provide a chemical crutch for those patients who seek help because they find it difficult to cope with the stresses and strains of everyday living? The provision of such relief may be appropriate in certain patients, nonetheless, what the doctor must realize is that he is curing nothing. In this context, however, it is well to remember that mental pains cause as much distress as physical pains. Their being less understood does not make their relief any less justifiable. Cure is also rare in physical disease.

Unfortunately, since treatment is symptomatic, patients suffering from emotional disorders have been sterotyped and categorized according to their check-listed symptoms. Furthermore, attempts to refine treatment in response to diagnostic labelling have led to additional stereotyping of patients so that chemical control over the charted symptoms of emotional stress is presented as a rational therapeutic goal. There can, however, be problems such as stigma created for patients who have been subjected to this categorization and labelling and yet these decisions by doctors are basically arbitary and their treatments empirical.

Perhaps for patients it may be better if they were not subjected to the hazards of medical labelling, provided someone helps them to recognize that often it is the life-situation in which they find themselves which is emotionally disturbing rather than they who are emotionally unstable. But who should help the patient to recognize and to rationalize his or her problems is a matter for debate. Whether the general practitioner is the most appropriate person to talk over the patient's problems (counsel) is something that no doubt this conference will be concerned with.

Nonetheless it would appear that the general practitioner will continue to shoulder the burden for the care of patients suffering from emotional symptoms, and if the recommendations of the Sub-Committee of the Royal College of General Practitioners' Working Party on prevention of psychiatric illness in general practice are acted upon then he is also going to be heavily involved in attempting to prevent these emotional disorders (RCGP, 1981). In the recommendations to this report, virtually no part of life's trials and tribulations is to be left untouched by medical intervention and we must surely ask ourselves whether such widescale medicalization is what is needed, particularly when we consider the socio-psychological implications of present trends towards massive unemployment. The report suggests that the general practitioner should be more willing than he has been in the past "to expand some of his energies in quasi-political activities". A learned profession whose members have not learned to cope with the limited medical model of emotional disorders now plans to extend its areas of involvement into what the RCGP report calls the socio-ecology of individuals. The thought of such an"iatrocracy" is awesome and perhaps after all, limited medical intervention, *improved to ensure the responsible use of psychotropic drugs,* offers greater freedom for the individual than the pervasive suggestions coming from the RCGP. At least patients have the freedom to exercise their own control over how they use these drugs.

We must, therefore, attempt to remain objective as "counselling" becomes the fashionable activity of the day. To use a reduction in the number of psychotropic drugs prescribed or taken as an indication of the effectiveness of counselling may be therapeutic to counsellors but what of the counselled who live their emotional disorders socially - is there any evidence that they do any better or worse under social tranquillization than under chemical tranquillization? The future

treatment of emotional disorders may well have to be a compro-
mise between chemical change and social change. Individuals
will require symptomatic relief (without the stigma of psychiatric labelling) and sensible counselling. The former could
be possible through the responsible and rational use of psychotropic drugs and the latter is not a special prerogative of
doctors. This does not imply that general practitioners
should not be knowledgeable about social and psychological
aspects of illness and about sickness behaviour (certainly
there is a great need for doctors to become more holistic in
their treatment of patients) but it does imply that they ought
to restrict their activities to being personal physicians in
the community with all the limitations that this implies.

There is a considerable pool of pain and suffering caused
by physical disorders and it is time that general practitioners
accepted more clinical responsibility for those many thousands
of patients subjected to the inconveniences of referral to
secondary care facilities each year. The need for such
clinical responsibilities is evident and indicates a need for
doctors to use drugs appropriately and safely whether in the
treatment of physical disorders or emotional disorders.

Finally, demand for medical intervention created by doctors
must not be seen as need. The important need of individuals
is for them to be able to understand the limited role of
physicians and their treatments in the community and to reduce
their expectations accordingly.

REFERENCES

Anderson, R.M. (1980a). Prescribed medicines: who takes what?
   Journal of Epidemiology and Community Health **34**, 299-304.
Anderson, R.M. (1980b). The use of repeatedly prescribed
   medicines. *Journal of the Royal College of General Practi-
   tioners* **30**, 609-613.
Austin, R. and Parish, P.A. (1976). Prescriptions written by
   ancillary staff. *In* "Prescribing in General Practice".
   Journal of the Royal College of General Practitioners **26**,
   Supplement No.1, 44-49.
Balint, M., Hunt, J., Joyce, D., Marinker, M. and Woodcock, J.
   (1970). Treatment or diagnosis. "A Study of Repeat
   Prescriptions in General Practice". Tavistock Publications
   London.
Balter, M.B., Levine, J. and Manheimer, D.I. (1974). Cross-
   national study of the extent of anti-anxiety/sedative drug
   use. *New England Journal of Medicine* **290**, 769-774.
Blackwell, B. (1976). Treatment adherence. *British Journal
   of Psychiatry* **129**, 513-531.

Cartwright, A. and Anderson, R. (1981). "General Practice Revised: A Second Study of Patients and their Doctors". Tavistock Publications, London.

Cooper, B., Harwin, B.G., Depla, C. and Shepherd, M. (1975). Mental health care in the community: an evaluative study. *Psychological Medicine* 5, 372-380.

Cooperstock, R. (1978). Sex differences in psychotropic drug use. *Social Science and Medicine* 12 (3B), 179-186.

Cooperstock, R. and Lennard, H.L. (1979). Some social meaning of tranquillizer use. *Sociology of Health and Illness* 1, 331-347.

Dennis, P.J. (1979). Monitoring of psychotropic drug prescribing in general practice. *British Medical Journal* 2, 115-116.

Dunnell, K. and Cartwright, A. (1972). "Medicine Takers, Prescribes and Hoarders". Routledge and Kegan Paul, London.

Freed, A. (1976). Prescribing of tranquillizers and barbiturates by general practitioners. *British Medical Journal* 3, 1232-1233.

Grimsson, A., Idänpään-Heikkïlä, J., Lunde, P.K.M., Olafsson, O. and Westerholm, B. (1979). The utilization of psychotropic drugs in Finland, Iceland, Norway and Sweden. *In* "Studies in Drug Utilization: Methods and Applications" (Eds U. Bergman, A. Grimsson, A.H.W. Wahba and B. Westerholm.) WHO Regional Publications European Series No.8. WHO, Copenhagen.

Harris, G., Latham, J., McGuiness, B. and Crisp, A.H. (1977). The relationship between psychoneurotic status and psychoactive drug prescription in general practice. *Journal of the Royal College of General Practitioners* 27, 173-177.

Hawton, K. and Blackstock, E. (1977). Deliberate self-poisoning: implications for psychotropic drug prescribing in general practice. *Journal of the Royal College of General Practitioners* 27, 560-563.

Haynes, R.B., Taylor, D.W. and Sackett, D.L. (Eds) (1979). "Compliance in Health Care". Johns Hopkins University Press, London.

Hemminki, E. (1974). Diseases leading to psychotropic drug therapy. *Scandanavian Journal of Social Medicine* 2, 129.

Hughes, E. (1973). Experiences of a general practice pharmacist. Proceedings of the Royal Society of Health, 80th Health Congress, Eastbourne.

Jones, D.I.R. (1977). Self-poisoning with drugs: the past 20 years in Sheffield. *British Medical Journal* 1, 28-29.

King, E. (1980). Sex bias in psychoactive drug advertisements. *Psychiatry* 43, 129-137.

Lader, M. (1978). Benzodiazepines - the opium of the masses? *Neuroscience* 3, 159-165.

Lader, M. (1980). Dependence on prescribed psychotropic drugs.
SK and F Publications, Welwyn Garden City.
Lennard, H.L., Epstein, L.T., Bernstein, A. and Ransom, D.C.
(1971). "Mystification and Drug Misuse". Jossey-Bass Inc.,
San Francisco.
Marks, J. (1978). "The benzodiazepines: use, overuse, misuse,
abuse". MTP Press, Lancaster.
Murdock, J.C. (1980). Prescribing of tranquillizers and bar-
biturates by general practitioners. *Journal of the Royal
College of General Practitioners* 30, 593-602.
Parish, P.A. (1971). The prescribing of psychotropic drugs
in general practice. *Journal of the Royal College of
General Practitioners* 21, Supplement No.4.
Parry, H.J., Balter, M.B., Mellinger, G.N., Cisin, I.H. and
Manheimer, D.I. (1973). National patterns of psychothera-
peutic drug use. *Archives of General Psychiatry* 28, 769-
783.
Pflanz, M., Basler, H.D. and Schwoon, D. (1977). Use of
tranquillizing drugs by a middle-aged population in a West
German city. *Journal of Health and Social Behaviour* 18,
194-205.
Raynes, N.V. (1979). Factors affecting the prescribing of
psychotropic drugs in general practice consultations.
Psychological Medicine 9, 671-679.
Royal College of General Practitioners (1981). Report of a
Working Party on Prevention Report from General Practice
20, RCGP, London.
Skegg, D.C.G., Doll, R. and Perry, J. (1977). Use of medicines
in general practice. *British Medical Journal* 1, 1561-1563.
Stimson, G. (1975). Women in a doctored world. *New Society*
32, 265-267.
Tomski, H.W. (1979). A survey of British prescriptions.
Pharmacy Management 151, 224-228.
Tyrer, P. (1978). Drug treatment of psychiatric patients in
general practice. *British Medical Journal* 2, 1008-1010.
Wadsworth, M.E.J., Butterfield, W.J.H. and Blaney, R. (1970).
"Health and Sickness: The Choice of Treatment". Tavistock
Publications, London.
Webb, R.C. (1979). Prescribing in Australia: Part 2.
Australian Family Physician 8, 242-253.
Wilcox, J.B. (1977). Psychotherapeutic prescribing patterns
in general practice. *New Zealand Medical Journal* 85, 363-
366.
Williams, P. (1978). Physical ill-health and psychotropic
drug prescription - a review. *Psychological Medicine* 8,
683-693.
Williams, P. (1980). Recent trends in the prescribing of
psychotropic drugs. *Health Trends* 12, 6-7.

Wilson, G.M. (1972). Prescribing for patients leaving hospital.
   Prescribers' Journal **12**, 63-68.

SESSION II
DISCUSSION

Chairman: Professor K. Rawnsley,
President of the Royal College of Psychiatrists

Dr Paul WILLIAMS (London): We are talking this afternoon about
one of the most important issues: the doctor wants to know
what to do. When talking about vocational training Dr Zander
drew attention to the distinction between knowledge and attitudes. Attitudes are important, not only in terms of the
individual doctor's attitude to his patients, but to quote the
WHO on psychological, social and pharmacological treatments
available to the GP: "transcending the importance of these
broad methods there are certain general needs, such as a
tolerant attitude, dependability, continuity and interest".
Attitudes are not only important in that sense but also in the
sense of openness to change, involvement in multi-disciplinary
teams, scrutinizing not only ourselves and how we prescribe,
etc., and also re alternative possibilities, alternative
models and alternative treatments. Clearly there is a need,
as Professor Parish pointed out, to demonstrate the efficacy
of such alternative models. It is also important that doctors
entertain the possibility that these new methods and alternative ideas may actually be useful.
    Professor Parish has sounded an important warning note,
that one can proceed too far in the direction of widening the
scope of general practice, so that we as doctors may believe
that we should have an answer to just about all of life's ills.
We must be aware of our limitations.

Dr D.W. MILLARD (Oxford): People's behaviour in practice is
influenced by their knowledge of the therapeutic potentials.
I am worried by the opening to Dr Zander's paper which presented us with a two-part model of the possibilities in therapy,
namely biological/pharmacological and psychological. It
excludes the third part, namely social adjustment.
    The use of methods of social adjustment is not, as Professor
Parish was suggesting, a revolutionary idea. Until the

nineteenth century most of the therapeutic potentials which
were available to doctors were along the lines of social or
environmental adjustment. We are all familiar nowadays with
powerful social acts, such as issuing a sickness certificate
which enables the person to draw money without working for
it. So I would make a plea for a three-part model of
management including social adjustment alongside the pharmacological and psychological methods.

Dr N. MISRA (Treorchy): As a teacher of general practice to
young doctors, Dr Zander gave an outline of the new brand of
general practice, including 3 years vocational training. But
by 1990 the GP will sit in his consulting room and advise the
patient to go to the relevant agency who can provide better
expertise than he can.

Dr ZANDER: Underneath the first question there is a fundamental point: "Is this whole business that we are involved in
for our own sake or for our patients' sake?" We need to open
our minds to other possible ways of providing care. But the
other point is also very important. In Israel are some eminent
medical schools. Of the first two thousand graduates from Tel
Aviv, Haifa and Jerusalem only 27 went into primary care. So
this very good medical training produced almost no primary
physicians. We must look at the effect of the vocational
training programme and perhaps modify it if inappropriate.
Having realized this problem in Israel, they established a new
medical school in Beersheba to train people with positive
attitudes to general practice.

Professor GOLDBERG: I was rather puzzled by one of the things
Professor Parish seemed angry about. He said that because in
the areas of unemployment the prescription of antidepressants
had risen, it means that a social problem has been medicalized.
I am not surprised that a social variable influences a psychiatric state. But if an unemployed Welshman who was severely
depressed consulted him, would he supply an antidepressant?

Professor PARISH: The symptomatic remedy is appropriate so I
would prescribe for the symptom of depression: but I would
feel very angry about the social situation. By medicalizing
it we somehow damp it down. We should guard against the whole
area of preventive medicine that the RCGP report recommended,
whereby you attempt to intervene in a predicted crisis which
would make for the breakdown.

Dr Richard FRANCE (Camberley): Two points by Professor Parish
puzzled me. First, those of us who advocate pharmacological
treatments do not merely practise social tranquillization.
Indeed, many of us believe in self-help skills, assertive
training, etc.

Second, we maintain we should be aware of the limitations of being personal physicians in the community. Some of the civic troubles in our cities reflect the fact that the city is a provider of services rather than a community to which one belongs. So we have this problem as to how far professional groups should get involved with social organizations.

Dr Andrew MARKUS (Thame): Prevention and intervention counselling are actually positive forces in that they help people to cope with their problems in future without going to doctors.

CHAIRMAN: A point raised by Dr Zander concerns me and the Royal College of Psychiatrists. It is whether the 6 months optional slot in the GP vocational training in psychiatry is a useful exercise or not, and what sort of experience the GP might extract usefully in that period? Could the reverse movement occur, whereby psychiatrists as part of their training spend time in general practice?

Dr Godfrey FOWLER (Oxford): That depends on the structure of the post. If the psychiatry post is primarily concerned with in-patient care it is inappropriate. If on the other hand it comprises out-patient and day hospital care, it is appropriate for general practice training.

Dr Robin STEEL (Worcester): Our psychiatrists have carefully planned their training programme, and my trainees have regarded the psychiatric 6 months as the one they have enjoyed the most.

Dr Timothy OWEN (Newcastle): The 6 months in psychiatry is invaluable provided it primarily concerns out-patients. One thing you learn is the proper use of medication.

Dr ZANDER: What is important are the objectives and attitudes and skills that we want people in practice to acquire. Some, but not others, are adequately achieved in one particular post.

Dr Richard VESEY (Warwick): I am a recent principal in general practice who has not done 6 months in a psychiatric post. It was beneficial for me to attend an introductory course run by the Marriage Guidance Council on counselling. I was with a group of people, social workers, etc. In 4 days I learnt more about counselling that I might have done in 6 months in a psychiatric post.

Professor A.C.P. SIMS (Leeds): Surely the aim of 6 months in psychiatry is so that general practitioners will be at ease in dealing with psychiatric patients both in assessing and interviewing, and in appropriate modern methods of psychiatric treatment including psychological methods. There is no basic distinction between conditions which occur in general practice and conditions which occur in psychiatry.

COUNSELLING IN GENERAL PRACTICE

Pamela M. Ashurst

Department of Psychotherapy,
Royal South Hants Hospital,
Graham Road, Southampton SO9 4PE

Jane Austen's Mrs Bennett might well have reproached her
family doctor as she did her husband - "You have no compassion
on my poor nerves". And most general practitioners could echo
Mr Bennett - "You mistake me, my dear, I have a high respect
for your nerves. They are old friends. I have heard you
mention them with consideration these 20 years at least".
Chronic minor affective symptoms have not changed over the
centuries, and literary examples closely resemble those
patients who present to general practitioners' surgeries in
this latter part of the twentieth century. Would Mrs Bennett's
doctor prescribe tranquillizers if she presented to him now?
I rather think that he would, for the management of such symptoms, although regarded as part of psychiatry's responsibility, is dealt with in the main by general practitioners.
Only one patient in 20 who receives psychotropic drugs on
prescription from their general practitioner is referred to
the psychiatric services, which have little to offer to the
vast number of patients seeking help for their discomfort and
distress at the surgery. Although increasingly psychiatrists
and psychologists are working outside the hospital setting,
the scarcity of this expensive resource and its basic separation from primary care makes it better suited to the consulta-
tive role than to the provision of continuing help.
A substantial proportion of minor psychiatric illness presenting to the surgery remains unrecognized and untreated, in
spite of the extent of psychotropic prescribing. Goldberg
and Blackwell (1970) showed, however, that even a trained
psychiatrist who had recently entered general practice and
was alert to the possibility of psychological disturbance
because of their survey, missed "hidden psychiatric morbidity"
which usually presented with a physical symptom to the general

practitioner. They found that minor affective illnesses seen in the surgery usually have a good prognosis.

A Lancet editorial (1978) reiterated the observation of Shepherd *et al.* (1966) made 12 years earlier, that a combination of drug therapy and reassurance was the commonest form of general practitioner psychiatric treatment, and noted that "in view of the high prevalence of psychological distress it is doubtful whether we shall see a fundamental change in medical management".

Advice and reassurance are an integral part of the help which the general practitioner is able to give to his patient, but their importance is frequently overlooked when new drugs or treatment approaches are being evaluated. Michael Balint (1957) described the doctor as the most frequently used drug in general practice, and many doctors have been influenced by his work in understanding the patient and his illness within the limits of the brief surgery consultation. Nevertheless, the extensive prescribing of psychotropic drugs in general practice suggests that many doctors resort to the prescription pad in cases of minor psychological distress, sometimes perhaps as a means of bringing the consultation to an end. However, Williams (1980) has found that the inflationary trend in prescriptions for tranquillizers and antidepressants, whilst continuing to rise, showed evidence of slowing down during the 5 years 1970-75, and the increase in psychotropic prescribing was less than the increase in prescribing as a whole.

Recently there has been a greater awareness of the hazards of dependency on minor tranquillizers, and articulate and informed patients, as well as their doctors, have been alerted by media reports and have challenged the wisdom of extensive prescribing for social and emotional difficulties. Is treatment appropriate and helpful in minor conditions which may be self-limiting? If the prescription pad is not the answer, what else can the doctor do?

During the past 10 years there has been increasing interest in providing alternative help for such patients, but few doctors have either the time or the skills to undertake counselling or psychological treatment approaches with more than very few. There has been a gradual trend towards delegation of certain aspects of work within a multi-disciplinary framework in general practice, and health visitors and social workers in particular may give much support and carry heavy responsibility for those patients who are coping least well with the stresses of life, or whose resources are seriously diminished, for whatever reason.

There has been much interest in counselling and a number of reports have emphasized the benefits of an approach which offers time for people to talk about their underlying problems

- a commodity which is scarce in the busy surgery - rather than a prescription for the presenting symptom.

Many doctors advise patients with marital and relationship problems to consult a marriage guidance counsellor and there are at present some 100 such counsellors working in the general practice setting. Waydenfeld's (1980) survey of 12 north west London practices using a counsellor shows that, although there is little evidence of a reduction in the doctor's workload or prescribing levels, counselled patients apparently derive great benefit from the service in improving their understanding and their relationships.

Anderson and Hasler (1979) reported their experiences of using a trained counsellor in their community health team. They found that it enabled some patients to reduce or discontinue psychotropic drugs even after many years, and that there was a reduced demand for medical time after counselling. Many patients were offered counselling help instead of medication, thus extending the range of treatment options available to the doctor. Only 13% of the patients counselled said that they would have preferred to continue to see their own doctor about their problems.

Counselling has achieved respectability in its own right, and non-medical counsellors may be able to contribute usefully to the "community psychiatry" of which the primary medical care team is deemed to be the cornerstone (WHO, 1973).

Evaluation of the effectiveness of the counselling approach has been based on a subjective assessment of outcome by the helper or the helped, and no independent follow-up assessment has been made. Counsellors show no great willingness to look at what they actually do within the counselling contract, and this also creates difficulties in attempting a rigorous evaluation. It has been widely assumed that counselling will only benefit a select group of highly motivated patients, and that medication is likely to be more cost-effective and beneficial to the majority.

During 1974/75, the Mental Health Foundation supported a pilot project (Meacher, 1976) in conjunction with general practitioners in the Hampshire market town of Alton, and in the London boroughs of Camden and Lambeth. Monitoring suggested that selected patients used the counselling service offered by 5 experienced non-medical counsellors, and that patients receiving regular counselling help consulted their GPs less and reduced their consumption of psychotropic drugs. The populations studied were very different: the Camden service was used by a mobile unmarried population, whereas a substantial proportion of the Alton referrals had a previous history of psychiatric treatment, and 89% of the Alton group were on psychotropic drugs at the time of referral to the counsellor.

The pilot study indicated, as other studies have done
(Reid and Shyne, 1969; Bergin and Garfield, 1971) that those
patients who improved with counselling did so within 3 months
of starting treatment. Unless they had shown signs of improvement by that time, most patients who were still being seen at
the end of one year made no further progress. Whether such
patients had simply transferred their dependency from their
doctors to the counsellors, whether they were unable to benefit from counselling help, or whether in fact they were in
need of long-term psychotherapeutic intervention was not clear.
How the patient group would have fared without counselling is
unknown. Because spontaneous improvement is common in cases
of minor neurotic illness, it is unwise to assume that change
or improvement is necessarily attributable to any intervention.

THE LEVERHULME COUNSELLING PROJECT

The pilot study findings invited further and more rigorous
evaluation, and the Leverhulme Counselling Project was designed
with this in mind. It has been based in Alton Health Centre
- providing medical care for the town's population of 18,000
- and in a city centre group practice in Southampton with a
practice population of 8,800 patients. Twelve general practitioners were involved, and 2 experienced non-medical counsellors, who had previously worked in medical settings. One
of the counsellors (VH) had worked on the pilot project. In
order to minimize the problem of counsellor effect, both the
male and the female counsellor worked in each centre, taking
referrals from all doctors.

The Leverhulme Project was designed to offer counselling
on a random basis to a proportion of patients aged between 16
and 65 years, consulting their general practitioners for
neurotic disorder, for whom a first or repeat prescription of
psychotropic drugs was given, or for whom such a prescription
was considered, or for whom counselling without drugs was
considered necessary. Admission of patients to the study was
thus decided on the basis of the general practitioner's
decision about treatment or management of the presenting
problems. The difficulties entailed in asking for a diagnosis
in an area which is intrinsically lacking in clear definition
were thereby avoided.

Random allocation of patients to the counselled group
involved taking control of the decision about counselling
referral away from the general practitioners, although they
were asked to predict whether counselling would be acceptable
or helpful to each of the patients. By replacing selection
with random allocation, counselling help was made available
to a group of patients for whom the general practitioners might
not have considered it on clinical grounds.

The number of doctors participating in the study meant that
there were wide variations in their approach to minor neurotic
disorder presenting at the surgery. Preliminary checks of
prescriptions had confirmed that the frequency with which
psychotropic drugs were prescribed and the quantity prescribed
varied considerably from one doctor to another. The inclusion
criteria were as broad as possible so that there would be no
temptation for the doctor to prescribe drugs in order to
enable his patient to have an opportunity to receive counselling help, nor conversely to withhold medication in order that
the patient should not be admitted to the trial. For ethical
reasons the project was designed so that the counselling
facility was an optional extra for the study patients, so that
no patient was deprived of any help or treatment otherwise
available to them. Although the random selection procedure
avoided any direct selection for suitability on the doctor's
part, his expectations of the counsellors, his knowledge of
the patient, his enthusiasm for the counselling approach and
his own relationship with the patient will all affect the
attitude with which the patient approaches the prospect of
counselling. Randomly selected patients in the group offered
counselling may fail to make or keep an appointment with the
counsellor if they have not found their doctor sufficiently
encouraging about the prospect, and in the event a substantial
proportion of patients offered counselling did not actually
receive it and presumably therefore found counselling unacceptable.

THE COUNSELLING APPROACH

The research design presented the counsellors with many problems, since counselling was offered to the experimental group
on the basis of random allocation, rather than to a highly
motivated self-referral group or those referred by interested
professionals. All 5 social categories were represented,
including patients whose approach to counselling was uninformed
and frequently negative. As the patient had gone to the
doctor to be "cured" there was an expectation that something
should be done to or for, rather than by, the patient. The
expectations of both patient and counsellor will inevitably
affect the investment which each makes in the counselling
relationship, and the outcome.

The counsellors were asked to make one major alteration to
their traditional practice, by limiting the length of counselling sessions to enable as many patients as possible to be
counselled. This also enabled a greater degree of flexibility
in the timing and frequency of appointments than would have
been possible with the traditional hour long session each week.

The initial assessment consultation was always for one hour and was used to identify problem areas with the patient and to offer a treatment contract based on an appropriate therapeutic strategy. Subsequent sessions were offered in multiples of 15 minutes, which could be increased as required, and at a frequency determined by the counsellor - a practice more in keeping with the doctor's surgery pattern than with counselling tradition, but one which placed unfamiliar strain on the counsellors.

A Rogerian approach was favoured by both counsellors, but the variety of presenting problems required an eclectic and flexible approach. Progressive relaxation was a technique frequently used, but supportive counselling, interpretative psychotherapy aimed at promoting insight, transactional analysis, behavioural techniques, Gestalt and dream work were all employed. The range of treatment offered varied in both intensity and extent, and was suited to individual needs.

RESULTS

The study population totalled 726 over a 9 month period, of whom 273 were randomly selected for counselling. Of these 157 (58%) actually made contact with the counsellor and received some counselling help. The total number of patients making an appointment to see a counsellor over a 15 month period (random selection for 9 months followed by a 6 month period of GP selection) was 267, and of these 254 (95%) actually consulted the counsellors. Information was available from 2 sources, the records kept throughout the study by doctors and counsellors, and the assessment carried out independently one year after entry to the project. Table 1 shows the selection for and acceptability of counselling in the study group.

Details of psychotropic drug prescriptions and the dates and length of consultations were available for all patients from the record cards. The proportion of patients in each group on tranquillizers at admission to the study were remarkably similar, with the exception of the GP referred group who were thought to be in need of counselling and not surprisingly were prescribed fewer drugs (Table 2). The use of antidepressants by group at the start of the project shows a similar pattern (Table 3), but more patients in the offered, rejected group were on antidepressant medication than in the counselled group. After one year, the number still on antidepressants or tranquillizers had fallen markedly in each group, but most dramatically in the GP referred group who were counselled. Those who withdrew from counselling were also more likely to come off medication.

TABLE 1

Selection for and acceptability of counselling

Met selection criteria	726	
Allocated for counselling	287	Not allocated 439
Excluded by GP	14	
Available for counselling	273	Offer refused 116
Offer accepted by patient	157	
Premature withdrawal of patient	80	80
Patients completing counselling	77	"Controls" 157

TABLE 2

Leverhulme Counselling Project
% use of tranquillizers by group

	Total no. in group	% on tranquillizers at entry	% on tranquillizers at 1 year
Counselled	88	52.3%	14.7%
Offered, Rejected	87	51.7%	17.2%
Controls	151	52.9%	19.2%
GP referred	45	31.1%	4.4%
Withdrew	82	45.1%	4.9%
Total	453	222	63

It is known that the length of time for which psychotropic drugs are prescribed initially is related to their continued use. Patients who are prescribed psychotropics for more than 6 months are unlikely to stop taking them. The number of patients on tranquillizers at entry to the study and at one year was analysed by prescription. The 2 counselled groups

TABLE 3

Leverhulme Counselling Project
% use of antidepressants by group

	Total no. in group	% on antidepressants at entry	% on antidepressants at 1 year
Counselled	88	30.7%	5.7%
Offered, rejected	87	46.0%	8.0%
Controls	151	48.3%	9.9%
GP referred	45	26.7%	2.2%
Withdrew	82	29.3%	7.3%
Total	453	176	34

TABLE 4

Leverhulme Counselling Project
% of patients on tranquillizers at 1 year
by group and prescription at admission

	Counselled Random + GP referred	Not counselled Offered/Rejected + Controls	Withdrew
Total no. in group	133	235	82
No tranquillizers	5.5	4.7	2.2
First script	3.8	7.5	0
R < 6 months	12.5	20.0	11.0
R > 6 months	38.8	48.2	20.0

were considered together, as were the 2 groups who were not
counselled. Five percent of the patients who were not on
tranquillizers at entry to the study were prescribed tranquillizers at one year, whether or not they were counselled. Half
as many patients who received a first prescription on entry
to the project were still on tranquillizers after one year in

the counselled group (3.8%), compared with the non-counselled
group (7.5%). Patients who had received more than one prescription but were on drugs for less than 6 months at entry
were similarly less likely to be on drugs at one year in the
counselled group. Of those patients on medication for more
than 6 months at entry, 39% of the counselled group were still
using tranquillizers at one year, compared with 48% of the
non-counselled group. Those patients who withdrew from
counselling had fewer prescriptions for tranquillizers in each
category (Table 4).

PREDICTION OF OUTCOME

Doctors were asked to predict whether counselling would be
(a) acceptable and (b) helpful to their patients at the
initial consultation, and before knowing whether the patients
would be randomly allocated to the group offered counselling.
Comparing their predictions with outcome, it appears that
doctors are good at knowing what will help their patients.
Ninety-one percent of those whom they predicted would get
better, did so, and improvement was well maintained at one
year. However, they were less accurate with their negative
predictions. Patients whom they said would find counselling
unacceptable, used it nonetheless. All felt better after
counselling and largely maintained the improvement. All the
patients whom they thought would not be helped by counselling
said that they were helped.

The counsellors predicted acceptability and helpfulness
after their first interview with patients more accurately
than the doctors, and were correct in their assessment of
outcome for all the patients in the GP selected group. The
records of prescriptions support the counsellors' assessment
rather than the patients' self-assessment.

DISCUSSION

The number of counselling sessions seem to make little difference to coming off tranquillizers, but the duration of
counselling showed some relationship to drug consumption, and
patients counselled for more than 3 months appear to have an
increased chance of getting off drugs. However, the patient's
state of health at one year does not appear to have been
influenced by the duration of counselling.

Counselling does not seem to reduce the demands on general
practitioners' time. Indeed, the more counselling that
patients had, the more time they spent consulting their doctors, and counselled patients used more GP time than the controls. However, patients selected for counselling by the

doctors used much less GP time than the randomly referred group, so the heavy demands of the latter may reflect a basic unsuitability for counselling and a need for continuing reassurance and possibly prescriptions from the familiar doctor. This interpretation is supported by the fact that patients whom the counsellors thought had improved, used less than half the GP time of patients whom counsellors rated the same or worse.

CONCLUSION

Preliminary reflections on the data obtained from the Leverhulme Counselling Project suggest that doctors and their patients find a counselling service based in the primary medical care setting both acceptable and useful. Counselling is not acceptable or helpful to all patients with psychosocial problems, but both patients and counsellors are good at judging whether counselling will be useful. Patients who reject the offer of counselling help, or who withdraw at an early stage, have a good chance of getting off psychotropic medication, and consult their doctors less than counselled patients. Patients who have been using medication for more than 6 months are more likely to get off it if they have counselling help, than those who are not counselled.

Patients who are selected for counselling by their doctors do well, and few needed medication or needed to use much of their doctors' time. However, some patients whom their doctors thought unsuitable for counselling accepted the opportunity offered by the random selection at the beginning of the project, and without exception they valued the experience, found it helpful and felt better for counselling, and the improvement was largely maintained at follow-up at one year.

Improvement with counselling was independent of the counsellor. The outcome for patients of both the counsellors working on the project was similar, although the working style and pattern of consultations was individual to each counsellor. This appears to have no differential effect on outcome, and the common elements of the counselling relationship are probably the most important therapeutic factors.

Those patients who were rated "very much improved" after counselling confirmed this in every respect. Counselling help made a dramatic difference to the lives of some patients, and a marginal difference to others. Although counselling is not applicable to all problems and all patients, and can never be as cheap to supply as minor tranquillizers, it clearly offers benefits to selected patients which make it a valuable addition to the treatment available in general practice.

Counselling may be effective in prevention as well as cure. Patients who do not want it will not use it, but there are plenty of doctors and patients who want it, who will use it, and who derive great help from it.

AREAS FOR FURTHER RESEARCH

The content of the counselling intervention warrants closer investigation. The quality of the interaction between counsellors and patient has not been explored. It may reasonably be assumed that some elements of counselling would be more useful than others for certain types of problems or certain patients. The elucidation of which elements for which patients and for which problems poses an important task for further research.

How much influence does the counsellor's personality exert upon the resolution of the presenting problems? Will all counsellors have equal effects? Can counselling help be replicated from one counsellor to the next? A controlled evaluation of common elements of counselling in a known context of practice would help to clarify the picture.

Our research suggests that the benefits of counselling are not dependent solely on the personality of the counsellor. Our patients did well irrespective of which counsellor they saw, and were equally likely to get off drugs and to maintain progress made with counselling. It is not known why some patients rejected the offer of counselling, and why some withdrew from counselling having made the initial contact. This area could be studied more closely with benefit, but clearly patients are capable of refusing help that they do not want, and our records suggest that they do quite well, particularly at getting off psychotropic medication.

If counselling help was available in surgery premises and advertised for self-referral, who would use it? Which patients would choose to take their problems to the counsellor rather than the doctor, and with what expectations?

It is a proper function of research to point new areas for investigation, more questions to be answered, and *how* and *why* would appear to be proper questions to further investigate the practice of counselling and its effects.

ACKNOWLEDGEMENTS

I am indebted to David Ward for his help with evaluation of Leverhulme Counselling Project data, to all the general practitioners who participated in this study, and to Valerie Hatswell who inspired and invited further study of counselling

in general practice. I am grateful to my secretary, Jill
Hatfield, for unfailing patience.

The Leverhulme Project was supported by the Mental Health
Foundation.

REFERENCES

Anderson, S.A. and Hasler, J.C. (1979). Counselling in general
practice. *Journal of the Royal College of General Practi-
tioners* **29**, 352-356.
Balint, M. (1957). "The Doctor, his Patient and the Illness".
Pitman, London.
Bergin, A.E. and Garfield, S.L. (Eds) (1971). "Handbook of
Psychotherapy and Behaviour Changes". Wiley, New York.
Goldberg, D.P. and Blackwell, B. (1970). Psychiatric illness
in general practice. A detailed study using a new method
of case identification. *British Medical Journal* **2**, 439-443.
Goldberg, D. (1974). "The Detection of Psychiatric Illness
by Questionnaire". Oxford University Press, London.
Meacher, M. (1976). A pilot counselling scheme with general
practitioners, summary report. Mental Health Foundation
Publications, London.
Parish, P.A. (1971). The prescribing of psychotropic drugs in
general practice. *Journal of the Royal College of General
Practitioners* **21**, Supplement 4, 1-79.
Reid, W. and Shyne, A. (1969). "Brief and Extended Casework".
Columbia University Press, New York.
Shepherd, M., Cooper, B., Brown, A.C. and Kalton, G.W. (1966).
"Psychiatric Illness in General Practice". Oxford Univer-
sity Press, London.
Waydenfeld, D. and Waydenfeld, S.W. (1980). Counselling in
general practice. *Journal of the Royal College of General
Practitioners* **30**, 671-677.
Williams, P. (1980). Recent trends in psychotropic drug pre-
scription. *Health Trends*, DHSS **12**, 6-7.
World Health Organization, Copenhagen (1973). "Psychiatry
and Primary Care". Report of Working Group.

SOCIAL WORK IN GENERAL PRACTICE

Roslyn H. Corney

General Practice Research Unit,
Institute of Psychiatry, De Crespigny Park,
Denmark Hill, London, SE5

Social factors have been shown to play an important role in
the causation of psychiatric illness. There is an extensive
sociological literature testifying to positive associations
between certain social variables and mental illness (summarized
by the Dohrenwends, 1969, 1974), the role of "life events" and
stressful situations has been investigated and discussed in a
number of studies (Homes and Rahe, 1967; Paykel *et al.*, 1969;
Brown *et al.*, 1975) while, more recently, growing interest has
been shown on the effect on illness of the presence or absence
of supportive relationships (Miller and Ingham, 1976; Brown
and Harris, 1978; Henderson *et al.*, 1978).

In addition to causation, social problems are often found
in association with illness. A higher degree of social
impairment is found in depressed patients than in normals
(Shepherd *et al.*, 1966; Weissman *et al.*, 1971; Brown and Harris,
1978), and chronic neurotics in general practice have been
shown to have a greater degree of social impairment than a
matched group of non-psychiatric patients (Sylph *et al.*, 1969;
Cooper, 1972). Although some of these problems may occur
before the illness, the clinical symptoms themselves - such
as irritability, tiredness and loss of libido - are likely to
put extra strains on personal relationships as well as affect
work performance and other social activities.

Social factors have also been shown to play a part in the
prognosis of mental illness, chronicity being associated with
long-term social difficulties. In a follow-up study on general
practice patients, Kedward found that those who had chronic
social problems were more likely not to have improved after
3 years than patients without chronic problems (Kedward, 1969).
Situational factors noted in these chronic patients were
severe marital disharmony, chronic housing problems, long-term
illness and bereavement. Kedward concluded that a great deal

of suffering could perhaps have been alleviated by social measures aimed at altering the patient's social conditions and thereby improving his mental condition.

In 2 more recent studies, the patient's social circumstances have been found to be the strongest predictors of illness outcome (Huxley and Goldberg, 1975; Jenkins *et al.*, 1981). Huxley and Goldberg in their study of 50 non-psychotic patients found that the patient's material and objective circumstances predicted outcome at 6 months while the investigation by Jenkins *et al.* on 100 general practice patients found that stress and lack of support in the patient's marriage, social and family life predicted continued illness after one year. Social supports may play a key role in determining outcome, those with poor relationships improving less often (Bullock *et al.*, 1972; Vaughn and Leff, 1976).

Clearly, social factors should be taken into account when the treatment of mental illness is considered, patients should not only be helped clinically but also socially. However, there is usually only limited involvement by the general practitioner in trying to change his patient's social conditions. This is partly due to the small amount of time he has to spend with each patient (Shepherd *et al.*, 1966; Cartwright, 1969; RCGPs, 1973) and partly to his lack of knowledge of social agencies (Jeffreys, 1965; Harwin *et al.*, 1970). Studies have shown that very few cases are referred by general practitioners to social agencies, including social workers (Shepherd *et al.*, 1966; Harwin *et al.*, 1970; Rickards *et al.*, 1976; Corney, 1979), suggesting that the social problems of the mentally ill may be neglected even though they may be important in determining clinical outcome.

This deficiency in service provision has been widely recognized and a series of reports and articles have advocated that the primary care team should be strengthened in order to give more satisfactory treatment to patients with psychiatric illness (World Health Organisation, 1973; Shepherd, 1974). These reports have supported the idea of attaching social workers to general practice so that they can deal with the social problems of the patients (Seebohm Report, 1968; Primary Medical Care Planning Unit Report, BMA, 1970; The Future Structure of the NHS, DHSS, 1970; Harvard Davis Report, CHSC, 1971). In recent years, a number of successful experiments on social work attachments have been mounted (Collins, 1965; Forman and Fairbairn, 1968; Ratoff and Pearson, 1970; Goldberg and Neill, 1972), and a survey carried out in 1977 indicated that over 50% of local authorities in Great Britain have at least one social work attachment to a general practice in their area (Gilchrest *et al.*, 1978).

Studies on the types of patients seen by social workers in general practice attachments have shown that high proportions of the patients referred have emotional and relationship problems especially women in the child-bearing years (Collins, 1965; Forman and Fairbairn, 1968; Goldberg and Neill, 1972; Corney and Briscoe, 1977; Corney and Bowen, 1980). Many are also suffering from mental ill-health, particularly depression and anxiety (Corney and Briscoe, 1977; Corney, 1979). These findings suggest that members of the primary care team consider these cases appropriate for social work help. The services offered by attached social workers include social diagnosis and assessment, counselling, the provision of practical help and liaison with other agencies on the client's behalf (Forman and Fairbairn, 1968; Goldberg and Neill, 1972).

Although the number of social work attachments have been steadily increasing, there has been little objective evaluation on their effectiveness (Hicks, 1976). Most reports have focussed on the subjective impressions and anecdotal accounts of the professionals and clients involved (Thompson, 1977; Williams and Clare, 1979; Corney, 1980, 1981a; Winny, 1981) and there have been very few independent assessments.

There are, therefore, strong grounds for evaluating social work treatment at the level of primary care using the scientific method of the controlled clinical trial. Although many have considered that they are impossible to carry out, a few clinical trials have been mounted in this country indicating their feasibility (Collins *et al.*, 1979). They do, however, pose many difficulties in their execution. First, there are the ethical problems related to the withholding of treatment to some patients. Secondly, there are the difficulties associated with deciding on which criteria should be used to measure outcome and on the instruments to be employed. Thirdly, there are the practical difficulties involved, e.g. patients refusing the treatment allotted to them or failing to attend for the follow-up interviews. Fourthly, there are the additional difficulties encountered when the "treatment" cannot be standardized or easily measured either qualitatively or quantitatively. No placebos are available, thus making a double-blind trial impossible. It is, therefore, not surprising that only a few trials of the efficacy of social work have been carried out on psychiatric patients (Weissman *et al.*, 1974; Cooper *et al.*, 1975; Gibbons *et al.*, 1978).

One study carried out on chronic neurotic patients (Cooper *et al.*, 1975; Shepherd *et al.*, 1979) indicated that it was possible to conduct a clinical trial in general practice. In this study 92 chronic patients from one group practice were assessed initially and then referred to a special experimental service which included an attached social worker. One year

after referral, they were reassessed and their outcome compared
to that of a group of 97 control patients referred from a
number of different practices in the same neighbourhood.
These controls were assessed twice in a similar manner to that
of the experimental group, but they received only routine
general practitioner treatment without the additional service.

The initial assessments of both groups were essentially
similar, but when the patients were re-interviewed one year
later there were marked differences pointing to benefits
accruing from the special service. Thus, the experimental
group exhibited evidence of clinical and social improvement;
fewer were taking psychotropic drugs; and their general practitioners reported that fewer needed continued medical care
and supervision.

In the light of the success in carrying out the study, a
further investigation was initiated to evaluate the effects
of social work on a more homogeneous patient population,
namely women aged 18-45 with acute episodes of depression.
This group was chosen as it has been shown to constitute a
high proportion of the referrals to attached social workers
(Forman and Fairbairn, 1968; Goldberg and Neill, 1972; Corney
and Briscoe, 1977). Research findings also indicate that
maternal depression has a detrimental effect on family life
and the children involved (Rutter, 1966; Wolff and Acton,
1968; Weissman *et al.*, 1972; Brown and Davidson, 1978).

The method used in this investigation is shown in Table 1.
The women were referred from 3 practices in a health centre
and a fourth single-handed practice a few miles away. All
doctors were asked to refer women aged 18-45 years presenting
with "acute" or "acute on chronic" depression. The duration
of symptoms of depression in the former group was operationally
defined as 3 months or less; in the latter group the symptoms
may have been present for a longer period but had intensified
in the preceding trimester. Women suffering from major
physical ill-health and those already seeing a social worker
were excluded.

All referrals were first interviewed by a psychiatrist,
using a standardized psychiatric interview (Goldberg *et al.*,
1970), and were then seen by a social research worker and
assessed by means of a standardized social adjustment schedule
(Clare and Cairns, 1978). Details of all those considered
eligible were then handed to a research assistant who allocated
each patient into one of 8 groups according to 2 categories
of age, married or single status and whether they were suffering from an "acute" or "acute on chronic" depression. The
first patient in any of those categories was assigned to the
experimental or control group by the toss of a coin, the
second patient was automatically assigned to the alternative

TABLE 1

Method

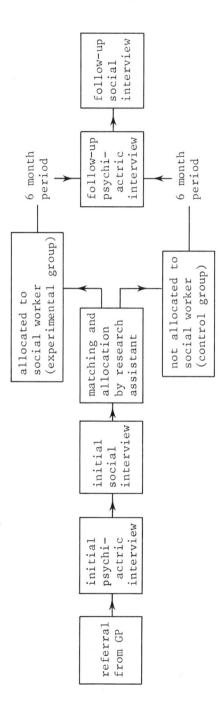

Data collected from the 1) initial and follow-up psychiatric interviews;

2) initial and follow-up social interviews;

3) medical notes for a 1½ year period
   (6 months prior to referral to 1 year after);

4) social work forms regarding treatment.

group, the third patient randomly allocated and so on. Those allocated to the experimental group were referred to one of 4 attached social workers for treatment, while the controls were referred back to their doctor for routine treatment.

After 6 months, the women were reassessed by means of the same instruments. They were interviewed by the same research staff who were unaware of any intervening treatment. Additional information was obtained by placing a card in the medical notes. The time of any clinical improvement or deterioration was recorded from the initial psychiatric assessment to one year later. Details were also collected from the social workers who filled up specially designed forms regarding each client referred to them.

Eighty patients were included in the study, 41 being allocated to the experimental group and 39 to the control group. Although 6 patients refused to see the social workers, these were still included in the experimental group, in line with the recommendations of Armitage (1979). The results were analysed by means of uni-variate and multi-variate analysis of covariance, taking into account the 3 matching variables and using the initial scores as covariates.

At the time of the initial assessment, the experimental and control groups were closely similar in respect of their demographic characteristics, psychiatric, physical ill-health and social ratings. There were no statistically significant differences between them. Approximately 80% of both groups were taking psychotropic drugs. Table 2 shows some of the initial characteristics of both groups.

The social workers recorded in detail their activities performed with or on behalf of their clients. They were not given any specific guidelines as to how they should work as the needs of the clients were remarkably varied. They were asked, however, to try to see their clients on a regular basis and to make a "contract" with the client, specifying frequency of interviews and a "plan of action" regarding their work in the following months.

Communications with the clients were classified by the social workers according to the typology developed by Hollis (1964). The social workers used "sustaining" and "exploring" techniques with all the clients they interviewed, investigating the reasons why the patient was depressed as well as offering support and reassurance. The social workers also considered that in 90% of cases, they tried to develop their client's awareness and understanding of the dynamics of her personal situation, behaviour and attitudes. In addition, the social workers tried to help the clients using "behavioural techniques" for example, helping the client manage her depression by

TABLE 2

Summary of initial characteristics
of experimental and control groups

	Experimental group (n=41) %	Control group (n=39) %
Married and cohabiting women	75.6	69.2
In employment	61.0	64.1
Social class I and II	17.0	10.3
III	68.3	79.5
IV and V	14.7	10.3
British by birth	87.8	89.7
Housing: Owner occupied	68.3	69.2
Council/rented	31.7	30.8
Duration of illness:		
"Acutely" depressed	39.0	48.7
"Acute on chronic"	61.0	51.3
Mean age (in years)	31.0	28.6

TABLE 3

Type of help given[1]

Type of help	Number of patients
Provision of materials, services, financial help	2
Advocacy/referral to other agencies	8
Information giving on practical issues	15
Counselling, discussion	35

[1]The patients could be given more than one type of help so
numbers add up to more than 35.

setting her a number of tasks to perform each day or devising
a "contract" setting tasks between husband and wife to increase
cooperation between them.

The social workers also gave some form of help concerning
practical matters to over 40% of their clients. This included
the provision of information, advocacy and the direct provision
of materials or services. Financial aid, material improve-
ments, holidays, day nursery placements and permanent council
accommodation were some of the items obtained either through
the social services department or through other agencies.

When the women were reinterviewed 6 months later, approximately two-thirds of both groups were assessed by the psychiatrist as improved (Table 4). Although a slightly higher proportion of the experimental group had improved, this was not
statistically significant.

TABLE 4

*Severity ratings at follow-up interviews
Experimental and control groups*

	Experimental group		Control group	
	No.	%	No.	%
Improved (follow-up severity rating of 0 or 1)	28	68.3	24	61.5
Not improved (follow-up severity rating of 2 or 3)	13	31.7	15	38.5
	41	100.0	39	100.0

The other differences between the 2 groups on clinical ratings
and composite clinical scores all failed to achieve significance.

The patients also made some degree of social improvement,
especially on those ratings measuring satisfaction, but there
was no evidence to suggest that the experimental group improved
significantly more than the control group on any of these
social variables.

The data collected from the medical notes revealed no major
differences between groups, either with regard to the number
of visits the patient made to the doctor or the length of time

during which they were taking psychotropic drugs. In addition, the experimental group did not recover any more quickly than the controls, and similar proportions were considered by their doctor to be ill one year after referral. Only a few patients were referred by the doctor to other agencies. In the 6 months period between assessments 3 patients in each group were referred to the psychiatric services for treatment. One patient in the experimental group was referred to a child guidance clinic for her son's problems.

In other studies investigating social work and psychotherapy, the results have indicated that certain patients benefit from the treatment while others do not, depending on the patient's characteristics or on those of the therapists (Fisher, 1976; Truax and Carkhuff, 1967). As this study revealed no major differences between groups, the data were then analysed to investigate whether certain subgroups of women benefited from seeing a social worker or whether there were differences between the social workers in determining outcome. Initial analyses revealed that the chronicity of the depression was an important factor in determining the outcome of social work treatment. More patients in the experimental group with "acute on chronic" illness improved than those in the control group, while more "acutely" ill patients in the control group improved than those in the experimental group (Table 5). This interaction between "treatment" and "chronicity" was significant when a multivariate analysis of covariance was performed on the clinical scores, and for 3 out of 4 of the "follow-up" composite clinical ratings. There was also some evidence of a significant interaction between "chronicity of depression" and "treatment" for some of the follow-up social scores and for the other indices of improvement such as number of visits the patient made to the doctor and state of health one year after referral (Corney, 1981b).

Additional analyses suggested that another important variable was the quality of the patient's relationship with her husband or with the opposite sex. Three-way interactions between quality of the patient's marital relationship, duration of illness and treatment were statistically significant for a multi-variate analysis of covariance and uni-variate analyses of clinical scores. When this variable was considered in conjunction with the chronicity of patient's illnesses, one subgroup of patients benefited markedly from being referred to a social worker. These were women with "acute on chronic" depression and with major difficulties in their relationship with their spouse or boyfriend. Of this group of women, 80% in the experimental group improved in comparison with 31% of the controls (Category B - Table 6).

TABLE 5

Number improved at follow-up interview for "acute" and "acute on chronic" depressed patients

	"Acute"				"Acute on chronic"			
	Experimental group		Control group		Experimental group		Control group	
	No.	%	No.	%	No.	%	No.	%
Improved (Severity rating 0 or 1)	10	62.5	15	78.9	18	72.0	9	45.0
Not improved (Severity rating 2 or 3)	6	37.5	4	21.1	7	28.0	11	55.0
	16	100.0	19	100.0	25	100.0	20	100.0

TABLE 6

Numbers improved at 6 months according to duration of depression and relationship with spouse or boyfriend

	A on C/Good rel. (A)		A on C/Poor rel. (B)		Acute/Good rel. (C)		Acute/Poor rel. (D)	
	E Group	C Group	E Group	C Group	E Group	C Group	E Group	C Group
Improved	6	4	12	5	5	12	5	3
Not improved	4	0	3	11	0	0	6	4
Total	10	4	15	16	5	12	11	7

Key: E Group = experimental group; C Group = control group;
A on C = "acute on chronic";
rel = relationship with spouse or boyfriend.

This difference was still present one year after referral,
when 57% of the experimental group were judged by their family
doctor to be well, in comparison with only 18% of the controls.
However, in contrast, women with an "acute on chronic" depression who had a good relationship fared less well in the experimental group than the controls (Category A), but there was no
difference in outcome one year after the initial assessment
(Corney, 1981c).

For the "acutely" ill patients, there were fewer differences
in outcome between the experimental and control groups; all
those with a good relationship improved (Category C) while
over 50% of those with a poor relationship failed to get
better (Category D).

Why did one sub-group of women (Category B) benefit from
the involvement of a social worker, while the others did not?
The difference in outcome could not have been due to any
initial differences in social scores (Corney, 1981c).

The patients who gained most benefit had been depressed for
some time and also had a poor relationship with spouse or
boyfriend. Many also had inadequate social contacts and a
poor social support system. Thus, the emotional support given
by a social worker may have helped these women more than those
who had good relationships and a happy marriage.

The social workers' records also suggest that this sub-group
of women were more "highly motivated" than the others. The
social workers assessed nearly 60% of these women as "highly
motivated" in comparison with only 15% of the women in the
other groups. This term was used by the social workers when
clients were willing not only to accept help but also to alter
their behaviour or situation accordingly. These women may
have been more highly motivated as they were receiving little
help from other sources but they also had more social problems
than those in the other groups. The social workers' records
also show that the social workers gave more practical help to
these women and contacted more agencies on their behalf.

Although women with "acute on chronic" illness and marital
or boyfriend difficulties benefited from social work intervention, there was no evidence to suggest that the social
workers helped the "acutely ill" with these same problems
(Category D). The social workers' records indicate that the
"acutely ill" with marital difficulties were less "highly
motivated" and many terminated their contact with the social
worker. It is possible that these patients were not ready to
accept outside help or regard it as necessary, having been
depressed for 3 months or less. Their degree of motivation
may also be related to their relative lack of social problems;
the social workers gave much less practical help to this group.

The results of this study – which suggest that certain
women might be helped, others harmed and the remainder unaf-
fected – indicate the importance of evaluating social work
intervention. The findings suggest that social work involvement is not an effective method of treatment for depressed
women in general and that it would be inappropriate for doctors
to refer all such patients even if the resources were available
The results, especially when considered in conjunction with
those of Cooper and his colleagues, suggest that patients with
more longstanding neurotic disorders will be helped more than
those with symptoms of recent onset. When the patient's
depression becomes "chronic" or "acute on chronic" there is
less chance of spontaneous recovery (Cooper *et al.*, 1969;
Kedward, 1969) and help from an outside agency may be necessary
to bring about any change. The patient may also be more
likely to accept such help and act upon it.

Patients with "acute" depression, by contrast, are more
likely to recover without outside help. The additional help
of a social worker may be unnecessary or even harmful, the
social worker interfering with the individual's own mechanisms
of coping or the support received from others. The patient
may also be less motivated to receive the help offered. This
is contrary to much of the reasoning behind the attachment of
social workers to general practice where it is considered that
social workers are in the most suitable position to carry out
preventive work (Goldberg and Neill, 1972; Bursill, 1978;
Jenkins, 1978) as it is often assumed that the earlier the
patient sees a social worker after the onset of his or her
difficulties, the more effective she will be. However, it
appears that *very* early intervention may be inefficient,
inappropriate or even harmful.

The results also suggest that depressed women with poor
relationships with their spouse or boyfriend may benefit more
from the help of a social worker. The lack of difference in
general between the outcome of the experimental and control
groups could have been due to the support the patients receive
from other sources including friends, relatives or the general
practitioner. These findings suggest that it may be the
friendship or emotional support which the social worker gives
to the client which is important rather than her technical
counselling skills or activities. In this respect, doctors
with sufficient time, health visitors, lay counsellors or
sympathetic volunteers may be as much help to these women.

However, social workers have additional skills and knowledge to these other personnel, regarding welfare rights and
local authority provision. The group of women who benefited
most from the social worker's involvement had more social
problems than the others and were given more practical help.

In the earlier study on chronic neurotics, where a substantial difference between the outcome of the experimental and control groups was found, the majority of the social work carried out was practical in nature (Shepherd *et al.*, 1979). Although social workers tend to stress their skills in counselling and underrate the practical help they can give (Wootton, 1978) it may be through their arrangement or provision of practical assistance that social workers can be of most help to general practice patients, including those who are depressed. Studies obtaining clients' views of social work help support this contention; all of them have shown that clients most appreciate the combination of practical help with emotional support (Butrym, 1968; Mayer and Timms, 1970; Sainsbury, 1975; Corney, 1981a).

It follows that future work should evaluate the effectiveness of an "attached" social worker with different patient groups and should specify the methods of intervention to be used or control for them at the design stage. The results could be used to guide the general practitioner on which patients he or she should refer and the social worker on the methods to use. In this way, the optimal use can be made of the social worker's time. Such work can be expected to provide a more objective assessment of the value of social work attachments to general practice and their effectiveness as methods of treatment.

REFERENCES

Armitage, P. (1979). The analysis of data from clinical trials. *The Statistician* **28** (3), 171-183.
British Medical Association. (1970). Report of the Working Party on Primary Medical Care. Planning Report No. 4.
Brown, G.W., Bhrolchain, N.W. and Harris, T. (1975). Social class and psychiatric disturbance among women in an urban population. *Sociology* **9**, 225-254.
Brown, G.W. and Davidson, S. (1978). Social class, psychiatric disorder of mother, and accidents to children. *The Lancet* 18th February, 378-380.
Brown, G.W. and Harris, T. (1978). "Social Origins of Depression: A Study of Psychiatric Disorder in Women". Tavistock, London.
Bullock, R.C., Siegel, R., Weissman, M. and Paykel, E.S. (1972). The weeping wife: marital relations of depressed women. *Journal of Marriage and Family* **34**, 488-495.
Bursill, M. (1978). Assessment of Social Work Attachment. Stage 2. Research Section, Kent County Council.
Butrym, Z. (1968). "Medical Social Work in Action". Bell, G., London.

Cartwright, A. (1969). "Doctors and Their Patients". Routledge and Kegan Paul, London.

Central Health Services Council (1971). The Organization of Group Practice: A Report of a Sub-committee of the Standing Medical Advisory Committee (Chairman Harvard Davis). HMSO, London.

Clare, A.W. and Cairns, V.E. (1978). Design, development and use of a standardized interview to assess social maladjustment and dysfunction in community studies. *Psychological Medicine* **8**, 589-604.

Collins, J. (1965). "Social Casework in a General Medical Practice". Pitman, London.

Collins, J., Cochrane, A.L. and Waters, W.E. (1979). An evaluation of social therapy in chronic alcoholism. *In* "Measurements of Levels of Health" (Eds W.W. Holland, J. Ipsen and J. Kastrzewski). World Health Organization Regional Publications, European Series No. 7, 209-213. WHO, Copenhagen.

Cooper, B. (1972). Clinical and social aspects of chronic neurosis. *Proceedings of the Royal Society of Medicine* **65**, 509-512.

Cooper, B., Fry, J. and Galton, G. (1969). A longitudinal study of psychiatric morbidity in general practice population. *British Journal of Preventive and Social Medicine* **23**, 210-217.

Cooper, B., Harwin, B.G., Depla, C. and Shepherd, M. (1975). Mental health care in the community: an evaluative study. *Psychological Medicine* **5**, 4, 372-380.

Corney, R.H. (1979). Preliminary Communication: The extent of mental and physical ill-health of clients referred to social workers in a local authority department and a general attachment scheme. *Psychological Medicine* **9**, 585-589.

Corney, R.H. (1980). Health visitors and social workers. *Health Visitor* **53**, 409-413.

Corney, R.H. (1981a). Client perspectives in a general practice attachment. *British Journal of Social Work* **11**, 159-170.

Corney, R.H. (1981b). Social work effectiveness in the management of depressed women: a clinical trial. *Psychological Medicine* **11**, 417-423.

Corney, R.H. (1981c). The Effectiveness of Social Work in the Management of Depressed Women Patients in General Practice. Unpublished Ph.D Thesis, University of London.

Corney, R.H. and Bowen, B.A. (1980). Referrals to social workers: A comparative study of a local authority intake team with a general practice attachment scheme. *Journal of the Royal College of General Practitioners* **30**, 139-147.

Corney, R.H. and Briscoe, M.E. (1977). Social workers and
    their clients: A comparison between primary health care
    and local authority settings. The Team - 2. *Journal of
    the Royal College of General Practitioners* **27**, 295-301.
Department of Health and Social Security. (1970). The Future
    Structure of the NHS. HMSO, London.
Dohrenwend, B.P. and Dohrenwend, B.S. (1969). "Social Status
    and Psychological Disorder: A causal inquiry". John Wiley
    and Sons, New York.
Dohrenwend, B.P. and Dohrenwend, B.S. (1974). Social and
    cultural influences on psychopathology. *Annual Review of
    Psychology* **25**, 417-452.
Fischer, J. (1976). "The Effectiveness of Social Casework".
    Charles C. Thomas, Springfield, Illinois.
Forman, J.A.S. and Fairbairn, E.M. (1968). "Social Casework
    in General Practice". Nuffield Provincial Hospitals Trust.
    Oxford University Press, London.
Gibbons, J.S., Butler, J., Unwin, P. and Gibbons, J.L. (1978).
    Evaluations of a social work service for self-poisoning
    patients. *British Journal of Psychiatry* **133**, 111-118.
Gilchrist, I., Gough, J., Horsfall-Turner, Y., Ineson, E.,
    Keele, G., Marks, B. and Scott, H. (1978). Social work
    in general practice. *Journal of the Royal College of
    General Practitioners* **28**, 675-686.
Goldberg, D.P., Cooper, B., Eastwood, M.R., Kedward, H.B. and
    Shepherd, M. (1970). A standardized psychiatric interview
    for use in community surveys. *British Journal of Preven-
    tive and Social Medicine* **24**, 18-23.
Goldberg, E.M. and Neill, J. (1972). "Social Work in General
    Practice". George Allen and Unwin, London.
Harwin, B.G., Eastwood, M.R., Cooper, B. and Goldberg, D.P.
    (1970). Prospects for social work in general practice.
    The Lancet **2**, 559-561.
Henderson, S., Byrne, D.G., Duncan-Jones, P., Adcock, S.,
    Scott, R. and Steele, G.P. (1978). Social bonds in the
    epidemiology of neurosis: A preliminary communication.
    British Journal of Psychiatry **132**, 463-466.
Hicks, D. (1976). "Primary Health Care". HMSO, London.
Hollis, F. (1964). "Casework: A Psychosocial Therapy. Random
    House, New York.
Holmes, R.T. and Rahe, R. (1967). The Social Readjustment
    Rating Scale. *Journal of Psychosomatic Research* **11**, 213-
    218.
Huxley, P. and Goldberg, D. (1975). Social versus clinical
    prediction in minor psychiatric disorders. *Psychological
    Medicine* **5**, 96-100.
Jeffreys, M. (1965). "An Anatomy of Social Welfare Services".
    Michael Joseph, London.

Jenkins, M.E. (1978). The Attachment of Social Workers to
    GP Practices. Research Section, Mid Glamorgan County
    Council.
Jenkins, R., Mann, A.H. and Belsey, E. (1981). The background,
    design and use of a short interview to assess social stress
    and support in clinical settings. *Social Science and
    Medicine* **15E**, 3, 195-203.
Kedward, H. (1969). The outcome of neurotic illness in the
    community. *Social Psychiatry* **4**, 1, 1-4.
Mayer, J.E. and Timms, N. (1970). "The Client Speaks".
    Routledge and Kegan Paul, London.
Miller, P.Mc., and Ingham, J.C. (1976). Friends, confidants
    and symptoms. *Social Psychiatry* **11**, 51-58.
Paykel, E.S., Myers, J.K., Dienelt, M.N., Klerman, G.L.,
    Lindenthal, J.J. and Pepper, M.P. (1969). Life events and
    depression: A controlled study. *Archives of General
    Psychiatry* **21**, 753-760.
Ratoff, L. and Pearson, B. (1970). Social casework in a
    general practice: An alternative approach. *British Medical
    Journal* **2**, 475-477.
Rickards, C., Gildersleeve, C., Fitzgerald, R. and Cooper, B.
    (1976). The health of clients of a social service depart-
    ment. *Journal of the Royal College of General Practitioners*
    26, 237-243.
Royal College of General Practitioners. (1973). Present state
    and future needs of general practice (Third edition).
    Reports from general practice, No. 16. *Journal of the
    Royal College of General Practitioners*, London.
Rutter, M. (1966). "Children of Sick Patients: An Environ-
    mental and Psychiatric Study". Institute of Psychiatry,
    Maudsley Monographs, No. 16. Oxford University Press,
    London.
Sainsbury, E. (1975). "Social Work with Families". Routledge
    and Kegan Paul, London.
Seebohm Report. (1968). Report of the Committee on Local
    Authority and Allied Personal Social Services. HMSO,
    London.
Shepherd, M. (1974). General practice, mental illness and
    the British National Health Service. *American Journal of
    Public Health* **64**, 3, 230-234.
Shepherd, M., Cooper, B., Brown, A.C. and Kalton, G.W. (1966).
    "Psychiatric Illness in General Practice". Oxford Univer-
    sity Press, London.
Shepherd, M., Harwin, B.G., Depla, C. and Cairns, V. (1979).
    Social work and the primary care of mental disorder.
    Psychological Medicine **9**, 661-669.
Sylph, J.A., Kedward, H.B. and Eastwood, M.R. (1969). Chronic
    neurotic patients in general practice. A pilot study. *Journal
    of the Royal College of General Practitioners* **17**, 162-170.

Thompson, K. (1977). Social workers have helped in care in general practice. *Update* **14**, 1401-1405.

Truax, C. and Carkhuff, R.R. (1967). "Towards Effective Counselling and Psychotherapy". Aldine, Chicago.

Vaughn, C.E. and Leff, J.P. (1976). The influence of family and social factors on the course of psychiatric illness: A comparison of schizophrenic and depressed neurotic patients. *British Journal of Psychiatry* **129**, 125-137.

Weissman, M.M., Klerman, G.L., Paykel, E.S., Prusoff, B. and Hanson, B. (1974). Treatment effects on the social adjustment of depressed patients. *Archives of General Psychiatry* **30**, 771-778.

Weissman, M.M., Paykel, E.S. and Klerman, G.L. (1972). The depressed woman as a mother. *Social Psychiatry* **7**, 98-108.

Weissman, M.M., Paykel, E.S., Siegel, R. and Klerman, G.L. (1971). The social role performance of depressed women: A comparison with a normal sample. *American Journal of Orthopsychiatry* **41**, 390-405.

Williams, P. and Clare, A. (1979). Social workers in primary health care: The general practitioner's viewpoint. *Journal of the Royal College of General Practitioners* **29**, 554-558.

Winny, J. (1981). Social workers have much to contribute. *The General Practitioner*, January 30th, 52-53.

Wolff, S. and Acton, W.P. (1968). Characteristics of parents of disturbed children. *British Journal of Psychiatry* **114**, 593-601.

Wootton, B. (1978). The social work task today. *Community Care*, 4th October, 14-16.

World Health Organisation. (1973). "Psychiatry and Primary Medical Care". WHO, Geneva.

SESSION II
GENERAL DISCUSSION

Professor Gethin MORGAN (Bristol):   We need to remind ourselves of certain basic truths about helping. Assessment
methods may lead us to meaningful diagnoses which in turn
guide us towards specific treatment and prognosis. Meanwhile,
the basic caring process is going on too, and the importance
of this basic process is often ignored. Recognizing psychological distress and listening to the patient are themselves
therapeutic. Furthermore, many of our interventions are a
process of playing for time, if we are honest about it. As
we ring the changes of drugs, or conduct counselling or psychotherapy, we are carrying out at the same time essential treatment of a basic nature.
   Dr Ashurst, Dr Tomlinson and Mrs Hatswell described their
impeccable study, relevant to the reduction of dependence on
psychotropic drugs, increasing perhaps in some cases demand
on the general practitioner's time by emphasizing the need to
select patients for this kind of intervention. Surely it is
not social tranquillization, because correctly conducted
counselling should give the patient a new-found degree of
self confidence and hope.
   Roslyn Corney coped well with modern technology and gave a
superb description of a very good study. She gave us insight
into the special problems inherent in evaluating social work
counselling, many of which I had not anticipated. The lessons
we should learn include the importance of supportive relationships, the importance of social factors in causing impairment
rather than in the aetiology of the original illness and the
need to be selective in our criteria of improvement.

Dr Alexis BROOK (Tavistock Clinic, London):   I should like to
comment on a few main themes.
   First, the issue that always causes so much discussion,
namely the role of the GP as regards psychiatric disorders.
To what extent should he limit himself to the medical model,
that is to look for specific illnesses to treat, and to what
extent should he adopt an "understanding" model? Professor

Parish has argued forcefully that we acknowledge that medical practice has its limitations and that we should, therefore, restrict ourselves to the medical model. Of course the medical model is of value: moreover many patients do not want to be understood, however much the doctor may know that they have psychological problems. They want their troubles to be seen as illness; they want to be given a prescription and resent it if the doctor attempts to give understanding. Having said this, we must accept that even if doctors want to adopt the view of only using the medical model, most patients will not accept this. Many feel very rejected if given only a physical remedy. Dr Zander has argued for an "understanding" model. I think that what he has in mind is something that is much more than, and qualitatively quite different from, what can be called the "traditional caring approach" that is usually adopted by doctors, and which is a blend of friendliness and sympathy, of reassurance and encouragement and the giving of commonsense advice. It is, however, much less than formal counselling and less than systematic psychotherapy. What he is advocating is what I would call "a psychotherapeutic approach appropriate to the setting of general practice". This approach has 3 essential components. The first is to try to understand the patient. The second, and the most important for the patient, is that the doctor gives him the good experience of feeling that he can be understood. The third, through giving him this experience, is that he can be "held together". Being "held together" enables him to feel that he can contain his anxieties better, and he is thus able to cope more effectively with his conflicts, even if they remain unchanged.

The second issue refers to training. Dr Zander stressed the importance of training in psychiatry as part of the voca- tional training for general practice, but questioned the value of the 6-month training in psychiatry given to a GP trainee, and Professor Rawnsley asked for comments about this. I should like to take up one aspect. Throughout his medical school career the student is taught only to consider the patient. He is not taught to consider himself, and how to cope with the anxieties that are at times aroused in him by the very fact of having patients in his care. With many patients the doctor has to combine trying to understand the patient, while at the same time having to cope with the feel- ings that the patient rouses in him. These include feelings of anger, uncertainty and, particularly, helplessness. Some patients not only rouse these feelings in their doctor, but act and talk in such a way as to offload them onto him, and if he is not aware of this he will find it particularly hard to know how to proceed. Medical school training does not

equip the doctor to understand and cope with these difficulties.
Professor Goldberg has described an interesting method of
training in this area which incorporates some aspects of the
interaction between patient and doctor. There is a need to
experiment also with other methods.

The third theme relates to the fact that many doctors,
whose particular interests lie in other areas, would appreciate
appropriate facilities for help with their patients' psychological problems under the umbrella of the GP's surgery. Dr
Ashurst, with Dr Tomlinson and Mrs Hatswell, has given an
interesting report on counselling in general practice. She
quite rightly challenges the popular belief that only patients
labelled "highly motivated" can benefit. Many are not motivated to look at their problems, but when given the experience
of feeling understood, not only feel "held together", but
begin to find that they want to consider their problems more
deeply and value the opportunity of being able to do so. It
is interesting to note that the time they allot for each
counselling session is more than the average 6 minutes the GP
can usually provide, and less than the traditional 50 minutes
of the psychotherapist. The 15 minute slot they allow seems
to be a realistic and appropriate time for a counselling interview in the setting of general practice.

The fourth theme relates to the attachment of social workers
to general practice. There are many different types of social
worker attachment to general practice, and Dr Corney has described an interesting experiment showing one way in which
social workers can work in that setting. Numerous attachments
of psychiatrists, psychologists, social workers and counsellors
to general practice are now being made. Each individual professional has his specific interests and characteristic ways
of working, modified to meet the needs of the particular
practice. It is important for each individual to clearly
delineate exactly what he does so that proper evaluation can
take place of the different types of work. It should then
gradually be possible over the years to devise the appropriate
psychiatry, psychology, social work and counselling appropriate
to the setting of general practice.

Professor Sidney BRANDON (Leicester): There is a danger that
we are going to concentrate on the good things that nice people
can do to those who are willing to let them. We have been
talking today about relieving distress and acknowledging that
between about 300 and 400 such distressed patients will be
generated by every practitioner in the country. We have not
heard whether attempts to relieve that distress prevent mental
illness. We confined our discussion on psychiatric disorders
in general practice to those aged between 16 and 65, if not

18 to 45. Many situations in children present a real possibility of intervention. But also we must be aware of the
demographic tidal wave of the elderly and the problems associated with them.

Professor John COOPER (Nottingham): What is the difference
between psychotherapy, counselling and case work in Dr Ashurst's
study? Many of the descriptions of what people did are what
most people here would call psychotherapy.

Dr Pamela ASHURST: Because we had people working at this who
regarded themselves as professional counsellors and we looked
at what counsellors did in this situation. We tried not to
interfere in any way with what they actually did.

SESSION III

PSYCHIATRISTS AND PRIMARY CARE IN NOTTINGHAM

John Cooper

*University Department of Psychiatry,
Mapperley Hospital, Porchester Road,
Nottingham NG3 6AA*

INTRODUCTION

This paper describes the early stages of a scheme to establish widespread and permanent direct links between consultant psychiatrists and the general practitioners and other primary care workers, in the catchment area of Mapperley Hospital. The scheme centres around regular (but not necessarily very frequent) visits by the psychiatrists to the premises of the general practitioners. This scheme does not involve any new activities or ideas, because this type of direct contact between general practitioner and psychiatrist has been well known for more than 10 years in many places. Reports of small scale short-term experimental studies, for instance, stretch back to around 1966 and 1967 (Gibson *et al.*, 1966; Brook, 1967; Lyons, 1969).

These studies, together with the programme of work carried out by the General Practice Research Unit at the Institute of Psychiatry (Shepherd *et al.*, 1966; Kaeser and Cooper, 1971) and the various studies and recent review by Goldberg and his colleagues (Goldberg and Huxley, 1980) tell us a great deal about the connections and common ground between psychiatrists and general practitioners.

There are now many examples available of co-operative ventures between psychiatrists and general practitioners. The scheme to be described here borrows a great deal from all this previous work, but is unusual in that virtually all the psychiatrists in the catchment area will be participating, and the existence of a psychiatric case-register will allow the study of any large-scale changes in the pattern of referrals from general practice to the psychiatric services.

Although some aspects of the effects of this scheme can be followed by means of the existing psychiatric case-register, it is not primarily a research venture. The scheme is going forward because it seems a reasonable and practical thing to do, and because a number of recent changes in the psychiatric staff makes now a good time to start. The scheme would be worthwhile even in the absence of a case-register, and the criteria for its success or failure will be the reactions of its participants, and whether or not it continues by common consent.

The general aim of the scheme is to improve the quality of the psychiatric component of primary health care. More specific objectives by which this general aim might be achieved can be regarded as a sequence as follows:

1. to increase the number of direct face-to-face contacts between psychiatrist and general practitioners. This should result in:
2. an increase in the knowledge that psychiatrists and general practitioners have about each other's methods and conditions of work. This should result in:
3. clear, stated and sensible reasons for referrals to the specialist psychiatric services;
4. an improvement in the quality of the psychiatric and psychological care given by general practitioners to patients they do not refer to psychiatrists.

The emphasis on quality rather than quantity should be clear. The main hazard of the scheme is that it could merely increase the number of referrals and have little effect upon their quality. A temporary increase in the number of referrals is expected, but if this continues beyond the early stages the scheme will obviously become unpopular and cease.

No apology is made for describing a plan of action rather than results. The scheme is still in its early stages of development, and it will be several months before it is working fully. If present plans are carried out, it may well be several years before there is any statistical evidence to show the effects of the scheme. Since this scheme can be regarded as a purposeful acceleration of a trend that appears to be developing anyway in many other places, it seems to be worthwhile to describe and discuss its early stages. Reasons for either failure or success will be of equal interest.

It is necessary to ask "Why is there a need for more and different types of contacts between general practitioner and psychiatrists?" Between them, the many components of the British National Health Service and the Social Services Departments probably represent the most comprehensive system of psychiatric, medical and social care in the world, and an

outsider might assume that sufficient opportunities for communication and contact were already provided. This may be so
for a small proportion of general practices and psychiatric
hospitals, but the experience of most of those who work in
the National Health Service suggests that there is plenty of
room for improvement in this area.

The reasons why a scheme of this type might be justified
are diverse. The first to be mentioned springs largely from
the education received - or rather not received - by the members of each of the various professions concerned (general
practitioners, psychologists, health visitors, social workers
and psychiatrists), about the activities of the others. Members of each of these professions often find that they have
surprisingly little knowledge of how the other works, and of
what type of patients and treatments they can handle. This
ignorance is not uncommonly accompanied by a degree of mis-
trust, particularly between social workers and general practitioners.

A second reason is that for every patient referred by a
general practitioner to a psychiatrist, there are many more
with broadly similar problems or illnesses who do not get
referred, and who remain in the care of the general practitioner. This was demonstrated some years ago by workers in
both this country (Shepherd *et al.*, 1966) and in the USA
(Locke *et al.*, 1965). These and other studies show that only
between 5 and 10% of patients identified by general practitioners as having psychiatric illnesses are in fact referred
to psychiatric clinics.

Studies of the reasons for selection of this minority from
the large potential group who might have been selected show
that the reasons are remarkably variable, and often do not do
credit to the health service. Fortunately, there is evidence
that patients with the more severe, resistant, and chronic
conditions have a better chance of referral to a psychiatrist,
but other points that emerge from study of this referral
process suggest that there is plenty of room for improvement.
For instance, when filling in an Attitude questionnaire,
general practitioners studied by the General Practice Research
Unit at the Institute of Psychiatry in South London gave pro-
minence to reasons for *not* referring patients to psychiatrists
which suggest that a greater ease of contact between general
practitioner and psychiatrist would be welcomed (Table 1).
The commonest reason given for non-referral is "the patients'
dislike of being referred to a psychiatrist", and a closely
related dislike to "being labelled as a mental patient" is
also well up in the list.

The opinion of the receiving psychiatrist about the
appropriateness of these selected referrals has not been

TABLE 1

Factors influencing against psychiatric referral	% of survey doctors[1]
The patients' dislike of being referred to a psychiatrist	60.0
A feeling that the treatment of neurotic patients is the job of the general practitioner	45.3
Delay involved between making the appointment and the consultation	40.0
The disadvantage to patients of being labelled as mental cases	26.7
The unsatisfactory way in which patients are dealt with in the psychiatric clinic	17.3
The lack of readily available psychiatric facilities	13.3
Consideration for the psychiatrists, knowing how busy they are	10.7
Lack of satisfactory rapport between GP and psychiatrist	10.7
Psychiatrist's delay in sending reports on patients referred to him	5.3
Others	10.7
Number of doctors	75

[1]Percentages add to more than 100%, since doctors often gave more than one factor.

From Shepherd *et al.*, 1966.

studied in detail. My personal experience is that about one-quarter of out-patient referrals seem to be unnecessary, but the experience and opinions of individual psychiatrists are likely to be as varied as those of general practitioners. In addition, but still at a personal level, I find that a significant part of my continuing out-patient workload consists of patients who need support or supervision of medication of a

kind that should be available for their general practitioner.
Unfortunately, when I start to suggest this, their response
is "I don't get on with my own doctor", or "my own doctor says
he has no time to talk to me", "gets very impatient with me",
"says it's just my nerves and to pull myself together", or
something similar. At the moment, for instance, I have 25
currently attending out-patients that I see personally. Of
these, 8 should, in my view, be supported by their general
practitioner. For the reasons noted above, I have not yet
terminated their out-patient attendances. I continue to see
another 3 patients because I happen to know from experience
that their general practitioners rarely follow my recommendations about medication, and its cessation would be likely to
lead to a relapse and urgent re-referral.

Finally, there is another and quite different type of reason
why closer links between general practitioners and psychiatrists
should be encouraged, to do with the need of the members of
every community to have access to a "healer". This term is
used here to mean our own equivalent of the shaman, ethnic
healer or wise-man so well known to cultural anthropologists.
Space does not permit the detailed discussion of this theme
in any detail, so I shall simply summarize a complicated subject by suggesting that the general practitioner is the direct
descendant of the local healer or shaman, and as such is a
vitally important and potentially powerful figure in the community. As society and professions have differentiated and
developed, some of the many functions of the shaman of pre-
industrial and pre-scientific societies have been taken over
by other professions, but a great many functions remain as
the responsibility of the general practitioner. Psychiatrists
have taken some of the more easily identifiable parts of the
general healer's burden of duties from the general practitioner,
but much remains. The growth of modern scientifically based
medical technology allows the general practitioner to find and
often to treat specific illnesses, but these new powers should
not be allowed to obscure the less easily definable role of
the general practitioner as local healer. Modern medical
education scarcely recognizes the functions of the general
practitioner to which I am referring, although recently there
has been some recognition of these matters in the form of
courses in medical schools under the arguable title of
"Behavioural Sciences". However, most of the more senior
doctors now working, in all disciplines, heard no mention of
behaviour (or communication) during their training.

One of the motivations behind this scheme is the assumption
that a "good" general practitioner or group of general practitioners will accept the role of "healer" in the first instance,
in the sense of being prepared to listen to whatever the patient
has to say, and then to accept some responsibility for helping
the patient to solve his problem whatever their nature. This
may entail obtaining the help of other professionals, or it
may not. These "good" general practitioners, however, certainly do not regard their job as simply picking out patients
with identifiable illnesses, either physical or psychiatric,
and dismissing the rest as none of their business.

THE TASK OF THE PSYCHIATRISTS

The activities of the psychiatrists visiting the primary care
premises will now be discussed. A list of possibilities has
been drawn up and agreed with all the psychiatrists as a basis
for action. The guiding principle is that each psychiatrist
will have to arrive at an agreement about what they do together
with the practitioner he is visiting, and that the activities
will be varied. For instance, they may be patient-centred or
subjected-centred:

Patient-centred activities

1. A full psychiatric assessment of a new patient by the
   psychiatrist, as if in a psychiatric out-patient department.
   This is likely to take an hour or more, and it is likely
   that the psychiatrist will make a diagnosis and start
   treatment, and wish to see the patient again in a week or
   two. That is, he will retain a clinical responsibility for
   the patient. The general practitioner may or may not be
   present during the interview, but he is expected to be
   present at the end to hear the conclusions and discuss
   treatment.
2. One or more the general practitioners may wish to present
   the history and present state of a patient, for comments
   and advice from the psychiatrist about how he, the general
   practitioner, might continue to manage the patient (or
   family). The patient may or may not be interviewed, but
   it is likely that the responsibility for action will
   remain with the general practitioner. This could apply
   to patients new to the psychiatrist, or to patients previously seen by him as in-patients, out-patients or in the
   practice as just described above.

Subject-centred activities

1. Most general practitioners have never seen a psychiatrist interview a patient, and are keen to take the opportunity if it is offered. (Neither have they ever seen each other in action, but this is another problem).
2. Either a general practitioner or the psychiatrist can take a common problem of mutual interest and introduce a discussion; subjects such as antidepressants, anxiolytic medication, psychotherapy, behaviour therapy, and the roles of psychologists and social workers, are examples.
3. Occasionally, a more academic subject and a more formal presentation or seminar might be given by either side, but this would be expected to be rare.

In addition, other professional staff from either the primary care team or from the psychiatric team can occasionally be involved. Clinical psychologists and social workers are obvious possibilities, and a joint discussion of various problems between psychiatric community nurses and primary care health visitors is another example.

It should be clear from these comments that the intention is to concentrate on personal contact and an exchange of information, as much as upon details of individual patients. My own experience is that it is all too easy to fall into a repetitive pattern with the same group, and after half-a-dozen visits of the same type, interest tends to wane. The intention is to keep a record of what goes on at these visits, and to keep reminding both the general practitioners and the psychiatrist of the possibility of varying their activities. There will also be encouragement to both sides to involve trainees in some of these activities; medical students, registrars and senior registrars are all likely to benefit.

Logistics

It is easy enough to design a scheme like this on paper, but its success or failure will depend upon how it is arranged and put into working shape: this in turn depends upon the structure of the psychiatric services and the disposition of the general practices. The current situation of these in Nottingham will be described so as to illustrate the practical points and problems that are being, and will be, encountered as the scheme goes into action.

Mapperley Hospital

Mapperley Hospital is situated in the north-east part of
Nottingham, and has as its catchment area the population of
400,000 or so which forms, for all practical purposes, the
town of Nottingham. A former physician superintendent, Dr
Duncan MacMillan, made the hospital well-known in the 1950s
and 1960s for a variety of developments in social and community
services. However, he retired in 1965, and much has changed
in the intervening 15 years. The Department of Psychiatry
of Nottingham Medical School was set up in 1971 and is still
entirely based there. Particularly relevant for today's
discussion is the historical accident that over the last 5
years or so there has been an unusual number of new consultant
appointments, almost all due to normal retirements. All the
present consultant staff are willing to participate, to
varying degrees, in the scheme, and some of them have already
had experience of similar arrangements elsewhere.

Consultant Staff

There are 6 consultants in general adult psychiatry, 2 senior
academic staff, 2 general psychiatrists with a special interest
in psychogeriatrics, one specialist in charge of the unit for
alcohol and drug addiction, and one psychotherapist. This
gives a total of 12 psychiatrists of consultant status to
take part in the scheme.

At various times over the last 5 years or so, 6 of these
consultants have had periods of visiting the premises of
general practitioners, so there is a useful foundation of
experience and interest upon which to build. Three have
already started, as a result of requests from enthusiastic
general practitioners.

General Practitioners

Two hundred and one general practitioners are listed as having
their premises within the catchment area of Mapperley Hospital.
Some of them work in Health Centres, some in small groups,
and some work alone. Table 2 shows the breakdown into those
in Health Centres, and those not. "Health Centre" is used to
signify premises leased from or subsidized by local authorities,
but some interesting problems of classification arise. Most
Health Centres are purpose-built and contain between 5 and 12
general practitioners and their teams, but a few contain only
3 or 4. The size of a Health Centre is no indication of its
internal organization; there may be 10 practitioners sharing
a building, but this does not mean that they work closely

TABLE 2

*Grouping of general practitioners
in catchment area of Mapperley Hospital
(Population = 410,000)*

Health Centres by total number of doctors and number of practices		Other Group Practices	Twos	Singles
Doctors	Practices			
2 of 12	2, 5	1 of 6	10	34
2 of 10	3, 5	2 of 5		
1 of 9	3	3 of 4		
3 of 6	2, 4, 4	10 of 3		
3 of 4	1, 1, 2			
2 of 3	1, 2			
Total GPs				
201(100%) 89(44%)		58(29%)	20(10%)	34(17%)
Total practices				
95	35	16	10	34

together, or even that they meet or speak to each other. They
are often organized as independent small groups of 2, 3 or
4, with no visible connections other than physical proximity.
Table 2 shows that 17% of Nottingham general practitioners
still work single-handed. A three-some is the most popular
arrangement, if independent three-somes within Health Centres
are counted (total of 18 groups of 3 = 54 doctors). There are
95 practices in all, adding together those in Health Centres
and those not, and counting the single-handed practitioners
as practices.

The Matching Process

An essential part of the present early stage of this scheme
is the sorting out and matching up of practices with the
individual psychiatrists, and I have concluded that it is best
done by one person (for the moment, myself). All the psychiatrists have provided their own personal opinions of general
practitioners they already know. Visits are now under way to
group practices to obtain their opinions and wishes about
psychiatrists they might wish to work with, and as far as

possible, suggestions will be made for initial contacts and
the start of visits which follow joint preferences. The
practices already visited have all been interested in the
scheme, and the only serious problems at this stage are practical ones of finding rooms and mutually convenient times.
However, I have started with some of the better practices and
no doubt objections will arise soon.

There are only 12 psychiatrists, so even if less than half
of all the possible practices wish to join the scheme, say
about 40, there will still be more than 3 practices per psychiatrist. This means that another necessary feature of the
scheme is that practices will have on and off periods with a
visiting psychiatrist. Some practices are already known to be
efficient and comparatively skilled in psychiatric terms
(usually containing our own Nottingham graduates). The intention is to start with comparatively good practices so as to
demonstrate that the scheme can work, and then try to move
into the less enthusiastic practices, helped by recommendations
from those already with experience of the scheme.

The time spent by the psychiatrists is agreed to be roughly
one session every 2 or 3 weeks, or its equivalent. For practical reasons, such as fitting in with general practitioners,
it is likely that most visits will be equivalent to half a
session, i.e. about $1\frac{1}{2}$-2 hours. This means that each psychiatrist will expect to make one visit to primary care about
every one or 2 weeks.

One important change in activity for the psychiatrists
remains to be mentioned. They are all being encouraged (and
readily agree) to cancel out-patient clinic time roughly
equivalent to the time they spend on primary care premises.
This will re-inforce the notion that there is no intention of
attracting additional work, but a hope of improving and
changing the present style of work.

Information from the Psychiatric Case-Register

Large-scale trends in referrals from general practitioners
can be followed on the yearly figures from the case-register.
The absolute number of referrals to out-patients and of
domiciliary visit requests are available for each practice,
and have been reasonably stable for the last 5 years or so.
The patients referred by each practice can also be characterized by their career through the services after referral:
for instance, some practices refer a large proportion of
patients who are only seen once, and others send larger proportions who are taken on for a number of visits. Some practices rarely refer out-patients at all, and figure only as
sources of emergency admissions.

Changes in these and other characteristics may well occur in the practices in the scheme, and would not be expected in those not participating.

Success or Failure

It seems likely that the long-term success or failure of this scheme will be determined more by user satisfaction than by statistics. If there is an excess of new referrals, the psychiatrists will rapidly lose interest. If the general practitioners find the discussions repetetive or too specialized to be helpful, they will begin to drop out in the medium term.

The scheme will be successful if, in about 2 to 3 years from now, it is still in operation and has gathered its own momentum for further extension and change, without needing constant monitoring and supervision. There is a precedent in Nottingham for this type of outcome for a collaborative scheme in the psychiatric services. The late Dr Duncan MacMillan arranged for every consultant psychiatrist at Mapperley in the 1960s (then about 6), to spend one session per week each in the offices of the local health authority, discussing patients and problems with the Duly Authorized Officers – a much missed body of valuable workers. All the psychiatrists did this and all enjoyed it, and it was almost certainly a major influence in producing and maintaining an excellent emergency and follow-up service, in close collaboration with these "Duly Authorized Officers". Times have changed, but perhaps we can be encouraged by knowing that co-operative schemes can sometimes be made to work.

REFERENCES

Brook, A. (1967). An experiment in general practitioner-psychiatrist co-operation. *Journal of the Royal College of General Practitioners* 13, 127–131.

Gibson, R., Forbes, J.M., Stoddard, I.W., Cooke, J.T., Jenkins, C.W., MacKeith, S.A., Rosenberg, L., Allchin, W.H. and Shepherd, D. (1966). Psychiatric care in general practice: an experiment in collaboration. *British Medical Journal* 1, 1287–1289.

Kaeser, A.C. and Cooper, B. (1971). The psychiatric patient, the general practitioner and the out-patient clinic; an operational study and a review. *Psychological Medicine*, 1, 312–325.

Locke, B.Z., Kranz, G. and Kramer, M. (1965). Psychiatric need and demand in a pre-paid group practice programme. *American Journal of Public Health* 56, 895–904.

Lyons, H.A. (1969). Joint psychiatric consultations. *Journal of the Royal College of General Practitioners* **18**, 125-127.
Shepherd, M., Cooper, B., Brown, A.C. and Kalton, G. (1966). "Psychiatric Illness in General Practice". Oxford University Press, London.

PSYCHIATRIC DISORDERS IN GENERAL PRACTICE – THE ROLE OF THE COMMUNITY PHYSICIAN

John R. Ashton

Department of Community Health,
London School of Hygiene and Tropical Medicine,
Keppel Street (Gower Street), London WC1F 7HT

THE PROBLEM

There can be little doubt of the extent to which psychiatric disorders are a public health problem. Some 89,000 hospital beds in England, equivalent to approximately 25% of all National Health Service beds are occupied by psychiatric patients and studies of psychiatric case registers such as those in Aberdeen, Salford and Camberwell are in agreement that about 2% of the population are in contact with the psychiatric services during any given year in areas with fairly well developed services (DHSS, 1981; Wing, 1971). The study by Rutter *et al.* (1970) of psychiatric disorder on the Isle of Wight concluded that a minimum of 6.3% of school children had a behaviour disorder of some sort if subnormality was excluded and Taylor and Chave (1964) in their field survey of mental health in a new town found that 33% of adults were troubled by one or more of 4 symptoms of minor psychiatric ill health (nerves, depression, undue irritability or sleeplessness). In Shepherd's survey of psychiatric illness in 46 general practices in London, 14% of a sample of 15,000 registered patients were found to have consulted at least once during the survey year for a condition diagnosed as largely or entirely psychiatric in nature (Shepherd *et al.*, 1966). In this study more than half the psychiatric conditions had been present for at least a year but only 7.5% of those received some specialist psychiatric supervision during the year. Shepherd found a positive association between psychiatric disorder and physical illness, an association which has also been shown by Eastwood and Trevelyan (1972). This association is important in underlining the potential role of the general practitioner confronted by patients

TABLE 1

The Epidemiology of psychiatric morbidity

Psychiatric beds (England) (DHSS, 1981) equivalent to 25% of all NHS beds	89,000
Proportion of population in contact with psychiatric services in one year (Wing, 1971)	2%
Prevalence of psychiatric disorder among school children (Rutter) (Isle of Wight)	6.3%
Prevalence of psychiatric ill health in the community (Taylor and Chave, 1964)	33%
Prevalence of psychiatric disorder in general practice (Shepherd, 1966)	14%
(Goldberg, 1970)	19.5%

TABLE 2

Some selected causes of death in England and Wales (1979)

	Number	% of all deaths
Ischaemic heart disease	145,253	26.2
Cerebrovascular disease	69,365	12.5
Pneumonia	51,250	9.2
Malignancy of trachea, bronchus and lung	32,890	5.9
Accidents (all kinds)	13,670	2.4
Suicide	3,943	0.7
Cirrhosis of the liver	2,004	0.4
Homicide[1]	373	0.07

Source: On the State of the Public Health (1979), HMSO (1980).

[1]Criminal Statistics England and Wales (1979), HMSO (1980).

presenting with physical illness and it has led to further
studies to measure the extent of undetected psychiatric illness in the community. Goldberg and Blackwell (1970) investigated 553 consecutive patients attending a general practitioner's surgery and found that whereas a general practitioner
diagnosed psychiatric illness in 19.5% of the patients, a
psychiatrist found additional patients whom the general practitioner had regarded as normal. These problems can largely
be covered by the labels anxiety/depression and problems of
living with schizophrenia continuing to account for a significant amount of the chronic morbidity (Table 1).

In prevalence studies as Taylor and Chave have pointed out,
"the size of the catch depends on the size of the mesh of the
net that is used" (Taylor and Chave, 1964). If the mesh is
small, a high proportion of the population will appear to be
psychiatrically ill, on the other hand, using a large mesh
and confining ourselves to mortality data out of the 555,000
annual deaths from all causes in England and Wales we would
be left with suicide which with 3,943 deaths in 1979 accounted
for 0.7% of deaths, cirrhosis of the liver (presumably to a
large extent alcohol related) which accounted for 2,004 deaths
(0.4%) and the 373 homocides equivalent to less than 7 deaths
in every thousand (Table 2) (HMSO, 1980a, 1980b).

However, as Mechanic has pointed out, the epidemiologist
relies on disease as the dependent variable and this immedi-
ately highlights the problems of psychiatric data (Mechanic,
1970). Epidemiological investigation assumes that the disease
under consideration can be defined and assessed, an aim that
is most convincingly achieved when definite pathological
findings can be demonstrated and which is least convincing with
the subjective phenomena of emotion. A wider view of psychiatric morbidity would have to include some proportion of the
13,670 deaths in 1979 which were attributed to accidents of
various kinds (consider the role of alcohol, of risk taking
and of reckless driving as a result of interpersonal crises)
as well as looking closely at the interplay of personality,
social influences and behaviour in the very high proportion
of deaths from heart, lung and cerebrovascular disorders
where lifestyle is all important. Taken together with the
more obviously psycho-social these conditions account for a
large proportion of general practice and casualty consultations (Table 3). In this very real sense housing, and the
environment, education, employment and recreation are legitimate areas of interest to anybody seriously concerned with
prevention. The connecting chain of causality between life
events which have their roots in the social and material sub-
soil and psycho-social morbidity have now been well described
in the work of George Brown and others who have provided a
sound academic base from which to work (Brown and Harris, 1978).

TABLE 3

The numbers of persons consulting or events in a year
in a British general practice of 2,500 persons

Conditions	Persons consulting per year per 2,500
Emotional disorders	300
Acute bronchitis and pneumonia	50
Chronic bronchitis	50
Acute myocardial infarction	7
Chronic heart failure and angina	45
Acute strokes	5
Hypertension	25
Old strokes	15
Severe depression	12
Suicidal attempt	3
Suicide (every 4 years)	1
Chronic mental illness	55
Poverty	100
Broken home	50
Chronic alcoholism	30
Divorce	3
Illegitimate birth	3
Committed to prison	2
TOTAL	755

(From Fry, J. "Medicine in Three Societies", Medical and
Technical Publishing Co. Ltd., Lancaster, 1969).

MANPOWER

In recent years the adoption of a community orientated philosophy of mental health has added to the pool of psychiatric
morbidity in the community. From a total of 150,000 in-
patients of psychiatric hospitals in 1954, there has been a
reduction to 89,000 today. This development has been in

keeping with the current commitment to community based care
but of course one consequence of it is to place a greatly
increased burden of work on community workers and in particular
on general practitioners.

GENERAL PRACTITIONERS AND PSYCHIATRISTS

The idea that general practitioners are the key to effective
provision of psychiatric care is not new. As long ago as
1958 a working party of the Council of the then College of
General Practitioners concluded that "every good family doctor
must be a good psychologist for psychological medicine is part
and parcel of all general practice" (CCGP, 1958). The report
went on to claim that:

> every general practitioner starts with an advantage over
> the consultant because of his knowledge of his patients
> and the background against which they live their lives,
> his accessibility to their families and the continuity
> of his contact perhaps over generations. He is the
> person best fitted to manage the great majority of psy-
> chological ailments....

The Royal Commission on Medical Education (Todd Report,
HMSO, 1968) stressed the importance of psychiatry in the
undergraduate curriculum and in the preparation of vocational
trainees for general practice and a commitment to the development of psychiatric skills in future general practitioners
has been a feature of the Royal College of General Practitioners.

In reality, the interest of general practitioners in psychiatry varies greatly. Cartwright (1967) found that general
practitioners belonging to the College were more interested
in psychiatry than non-members and May and Gregory (1968)
found that among 69 randomly sampled general practitioners
those who had undergone some postgraduate psychiatric training
seemed to be in a position to make a much more positive contribution (May and Gregory, 1968). Mowbray *et al.* (1961) in
a study of members of the College of General Practitioners
concluded that only a minority were especially interested in
psychiatry. It is studies such as these which have convinced
Johnson (Johnson, 1973, 1974) that the lack of interest shown
by general practitioners in psychiatry makes it unrealistic
to base psychiatric care on them. It is to be hoped that such
conclusions are pessimistic in view of the growing strength
of postgraduate training in general practice and the recent
College initiative in preventive psychiatry (RCGP, 1981).

Unfortunately, even if a general practitioner has a special
interest in psychiatry, he would be hard put to deal adequately

with the psychiatric morbidity in his practice. Kessel (1965)
has concluded that if a doctor tried to see each psychologically
disturbed patient on his list for 10 minutes each month, this
would involve him in 14 hours a week in addition to his other
work. General practitioners faced with even the overt morbidity amongst their patients are likely to resort to pharmacological treatments as the simplest choice.

The provision of an adequate, appropriate and equal psychiatric service would appear to require an emphasis on community provision. It is likely that when interested, general
practitioners can play a major part in providing this service
together with other members of primary health care and social
services teams supported by psychiatrists. However, relying
on the whim and interest of individuals is no way to provide
a uniform service and the difficulty of interesting all general
practitioners in psychiatry on the one hand and all psychiatrists in the community on the other, poses major obstacles.
Aldrich (1965) has claimed that the psychiatrist of the future
will:

> give a much greater part of his time to teaching and
> consulting with physicians, psychologists, social work-
> ers, nurses, health visitors, clergymen, probation
> officers, teachers in special schools and others in
> direct contact with emotionally disturbed patients out-
> side psychiatric settings.

There is little to suggest that this imaginative concept of
psychiatry is a generally held self-perception of psychiatrists.
It is a depressing reality that when psychiatrists talk of
prevention they almost inevitably mean early diagnosis and
physical treatment.

THE COMMUNITY PHYSICIAN

Since 1974 it has been the job of the community physician to
take an overview, to plan for the efficient and effective
delivery of medical services and to address the challenge of
prevention. Who is this person and what does he actually
do?

The community physician is in fact the metamorphosis of the
Medical Officer of Health - a doctor usually a man who had his
origins in the appalling environmental problems of the industrial towns 150 years ago. At that time, epidemics of infectious disease thrived on malnourished populations living in
slum dwellings and in poverty. Male life expectancy at birth
was 40 years and up to a quarter of infants failed to see their
first birthday. In his classic "Report on the Sanitary Condition of the Labouring Population", Chadwick made the case for

the appointment of a District Medical Officer independent of private practice and responsible for the prevention of disease to be the advocate of the public health. He was to tackle the fundamental threats to the public health at that time (Chadwick, 1842). Eventually such Medical Officers of Health were appointed throughout the country and the ensuing battles of the sanitary and public health revolutions are well documented (Chave, SPW, 1980). By the 1930s, the Medical Officer of Health had an established reputation and a strong local authority team to back him up.

The advent of the National Health Service with its tri-partite structure of hospitals, general practice and community health services, led to the separation of preventive and curative medicine. Ironically this was at a time when it was becoming increasingly clear that there was a need for a "modern public health" to develop new methods of prevention for the behaviour-based diseases of the present as opposed to the infectious diseases of the past. Simultaneously, the escalating costs of medical care led to the recognition of the need for planning in the health service to enable scarce resources to be put to their best use.

In 1969 in a seminal paper, Professor Morris described the role of a new public health doctor as "The Community Physician" (Morris, 1969). This person was to be a doctor who was trained in epidemiology, statistics and the behavioural sciences (Table 4); his focus would be the health of a defined population rather than the sickness of specific individuals. His training would equip him to take a comprehensive view of health and disease, to act as an administrator of local ser-vices, epidemiologist and community counsellor and to develop strategies of health promotion and disease prevention for the population for which he was responsible (Table 5). These functions were all seen to be applications of the uses of epidemiology (Table 6).

The idea of the community physician took root and at the re-organization of the NHS in 1974 the new doctor came into existence. In the grey book outlining the arrangements for the re-organized health service, his job was described as "a specialist .... an accountable manager and as an adviser to and a manager of services for local government ...." (HMSO, 1972). His roles were to include planning, developing and interpreting information, evaluating service effectiveness and co-ordinating preventive care services.

In the developing policies of community care for psychiatry one would have expected that the community physician would be about to play a major co-ordinating and planning role. How-ever, from a review of the subsequent literature one might be

TABLE 4

*The syllabus of the M.Sc. degree in Community Medicine
at the London School of Hygiene and Tropical Medicine*

1. Epidemiology.

2. Statistics, survey methods, operational research, computing.

3. Vital statistics and health information systems.

4. The organization of medical care.

5. Social and behavioural sciences (sociology, social policy
   and social administration, organizations theory, health
   economics).

6. Preventive medicine and health education.

7. Acute community medicine, infectious disease, environmental health.

8. Special client groups; mental health, maternal and child
   care, the elderly, etc.

9. Principles of administration and management.

TABLE 5

Public health approach to prevention

1. Primary prevention:

   Health promotion and the removal of influences
   causing ill health.

2. Secondary prevention:

   Early diagnosis and appropriate treatment.

3. Tertiary prevention:

   Rehabilitation.

forgiven for thinking that his course has been downhill ever
since (Hall and Donaldson, 1979). Poor recruitment, role
confusion with an apparent preoccupation with routine administration and an indifferent reception from clinical colleagues
appear to have characterized his career so far. However, the
reality is that the nature of modern health problems must mean
that the community physician is here to stay; the advances to

TABLE 6

The uses of epidemiology

---

1. To study the history of the health of populations.

2. To diagnose the health of the community.

3. To study the working of health services.

4. To estimate the individual risks based on group experiences.

5. To identify syndromes by describing the distribution and association of clinical phenomena in the population.

6. To complete the clinical picture and describe the natural history.

7. To search for causes.

(From Morris, J.N. "The Uses of Epidemiology". Churchill Livingstone, 1975).

be made from a technological and treatment orientated approach are increasingly seen as extremely limited whilst the preventable nature of a great deal of morbidity is now apparent. The work of the community physician is likely to become more, not less important and in the view of a growing number of those in the field the sooner he retrieves his preventive brief, the more likely he is to make a contribution to the public health (Griffiths *et al.*, 1981).

WHAT IS TO BE DONE?

The picture painted so far in this paper is a depressing one, albeit perhaps a caricature - psychiatrists who rarely venture out from the safety of their hospitals, general practitioners with a variable interest in prevention of any kind, let alone that of mental ill health and finally community physicians who are understrength, under-resourced and losing morale.

All this against a backcloth of the worst economic recession for 50 years where the traditional public health problems associated with unemployment and poverty seem likely to return and where reduced investment in state education prevents any possibility of effective education for living and for positive health. The diseases of affluence and those of poverty are beginning to meet but going backwards - alcohol is now back on the agenda in a big way.

Whatever the answer to this new public health challenge it is clear that no one person or professional group can do it

alone. There *are* no more heroes. Doctors, whether they like
it or not have to work together with many other different
types of people – not only nurses, health visitors, social
workers, and therapists of various kinds but also health
education officers, local government officials, politicians
and volunteers, even the media. Draper and his colleagues
have argued eloquently the need for a new approach in public
health based on the development of multi-disciplinary health
promotion teams operating at the different levels at which
action is appropriate (Table 7) (Draper *et al.*, 1979; Griffiths
et al., 1981). It is anticipated that these teams will tackle
the major policy issues at national and local level by acting
on the political process, the organizational issues at
national, regional and local level by addressing their work
to the appropriate institutions, and the individual issues
through the development of a non-victim blaming approach to
health education aimed at demystifying medicine and involving
the people in maintaining and promoting their own health.

TABLE 7

*A model for prevention strategies related to
specific public health problems*

Level of prevention	Level of action		
	Policy	Organizational	Individual
Primary			
Secondary			
Tertiary			

The time in many ways seems ripe for such a development.
The problems are here and upon us. Traditional approaches
based on 1:1 treatment, increasingly seem bankrupt or prohibi-
tively expensive; prevention has become the slogan of all
parties.

Despite the pessimistic note of the early part of this
paper, there is growing interest in epidemiology as a tool of
prevention amongst both hospital clinicians and general practitioners. Short courses of epidemiology provided for these
groups are inevitably grossly over-subscribed. The Royal
College of Psychiatrists Report on Alcoholism was a most welcome initiative (RCPsych., 1979). In general practice the
work of the College over the past 15 years has established the
groundwork for a potentially fruitful future - new general
practitioners are technically competent over a wide area of
practice. Through the influence of Balint and Byrne they are
much more likely than formerly to be in a position to see
things from the patient's point of view (Balint, 1957; Byrne
and Long, 1976). Increasingly they practise from high quality
premises as members of a multi-disciplinary group which is
potentially a team. Most important of all and unusually
among western countries general practitioners have a defined
list - they know who their population is, who they are responsible for, the denominator of the public health equation.
What is needed now is the conceptual and functional leap
implicit in the 1974 reorganization towards an integrated
population view of clinical practice and prevention. Clinical
teams need to see the health district population or the practice list as the population for which they are responsible and
not just the patients who knock on the door. The focus of
interest must extend out from the institution whether it be
hospital or health centre to the elements of the community
productive of health and illness. (Housing, factories and
offices, the environment, social and recreational institutions
- the structures and what goes on within them.) It must come
to be seen as part of the legitimate work of teams to be pro-
active; to initiate action at political, organizational or
individual level - in a way the village doctor always had this
capacity.

The models of Will Pickles and of Chadwick remain apposite
(Pickles, 1972). If Pickles were alive today I believe he
would have an age-sex register and a morbidity index which not
only existed but which would be used on an operational basis
to identify what needed to be done and where. If Chadwick
were alive he would have priorities which included alcohol,
smoking, accident prevention, diet and exercise; sadly, living
and working conditions would still have to be high on his
list and the Brewers would be in for a rough time. He would

not have taken the cuts in education and school meals lying down but would have pointed out that in the long term they would prove more expensive both in pure economic terms and also in terms of the harvest of social and clinical pathology to be reaped. In a society of great social and geographical mobility where child care was increasingly based on small nuclear units and single parent households, I believe Chadwick would have argued the case for nursery education and child benefit every bit as strongly and along the same utilitarian lines. Today it is the Community Physicians' task to enable this to happen and to provide the information for the debate, not as a hero but as a catalyst to the many and increasing pro-health forces. The development of epidemiology teaching and seminars, of appropriate information systems based on the age-sex register at general practice level, on relevant hospital out-patient and in-patient activity analyses and on social services data, together with *ad hoc* surveys as necessary are a prerequisite for the logical operation of health promotion. It is for the community physician to enable their development and it is for him to bring the various teams together. It is on his ability to act as a catalyst in this sense that the community physician will be judged. What is needed is a dissemination of epidemiological thinking as a basis for collective action, a conceptual framework within which to operate, and the effective operation of teams by which to achieve our goal - to improve the health of the people.

ACKNOWLEDGEMENT

Parts of this paper have previously appeared in Update (February 1st, 1979, p.313-318) under the title "The GP's Role in Psychiatric Care".

REFERENCES

Aldrich, C.K. (1965). Psychiatric consultation in general practice. *Lancet* i, 805.
Balint, M. (1957). "The Doctor, his Patient and the Illness". Pitman Medical, London.
Brown, G.W. and Harris, T.O. (1978). "The Social Origins of Depression". Tavistock, London.
Byrne, P.S. and Long, B.E.L. (1976). "Doctors Talking to Patients". HMSO, London.
Cartwright, A. (1967). "Patients and their Doctors". Routledge and Kegan Paul, London.

Chadwick, E. (1842). Report on the Sanitary Condition of the Labouring Population of Great Britain. Resume in "Documents on Health and Social Services, 1834 to the Present Day". Brian Watkin, Methuen and Co., 1975.

Chave, S.P.W. (1980). The rise and fall of the medical officer of health. *Community Medicine* **2**, 36-45.

Council of College of General Practitioners (1958). Psychological medicine in general practice. *British Medical Journal* **2**, 585.

DHSS (1981). SH$_3$ National Summary for 1979 (England) (unpublished data).

Draper, P. (1979). "Rethinking Community Medicine: Towards a Renaissance in Public Health". USHP, London.

Eastwood, M.R. and Trevelyan, M.H. (1972). Relation between physical and psychiatric disorders. *Psychological Medicine* ii, 362-372.

Fry, J. (1969). "Medicine in Three Societies". Medical and Technical Publishing Co. Ltd., Lancaster.

Goldberg, D.P. and Blackwell, B. (1970). Psychiatric illness in general practice: a detailed study using a new method of case identification. *British Medical Journal* **2**, 439.

Griffiths, J., Dennis, J. and Draper, P. (1981). Prevention and the community physician. *In* "Recent Advances in Community Medicine. 2". Churchill Livingstone, London.

Hall, D.J. and Donaldson, R.J. (1979). A comparison of the work of doctors in community medicine in the United Kingdom. *Community Medicine* **1**, 137-152.

HMSO (1968). The Royal Commission on Medical Education (Todd Report).

HMSO (1972). Management Arrangements for the Reorganized National Health Service.

HMSO (1980a). Criminal Statistics England and Wales (1979).

HMSO (1980b). On the State of the Public Health for the year 1979.

Johnson, D.A.W. (1973a). Treatment of depression in general practice. *British Medical Journal* **2**, 18-20.

Johnson, D.A.W. (1974). A study of the use of antidepressant medication in general practice. *British Journal of Psychiatry* **125**, 186-192.

Kessel, N. (1965). The neurotic in general practice. *Practitioner* **194**, 636-641.

May, A.R. and Gregory, E. (1968). Participation of general practitioners in community psychiatry. *British Medical Journal* **2**, 168-171.

Mechanic, D. (1970). Problems and prospects in psychiatric epidemiology. *In* "An International Symposium of Psychiatric Epidemiology". (Eds E.H. Hare and J.K. Wing). Nuffield Provincial Hospitals Trust and Oxford University Press.

Morris, J.N. (1975). "The Uses of Epidemiology". Churchill
Livingstone, London.
Morris, J.N. (1969). Tomorrow's community physician. *Lancet*
ii, 811.
Mowbray, R.M., Blair, W., Jubb, L.G. and Clarke, A. (1961).
The general practitioner's attitude to psychiatry.
Scottish Medical Journal **6**, 314.
Pickles, W.N. (1972). "Epidemiology in Country Practice".
The Devonshire Press.
RCPsych. (1979). Alcohol and Alcoholism. The Report of a
Special Committee of the Royal College of Psychiatrists.
Tavistock Publications.
Royal College of General Practitioners (1981). Prevention of
Psychiatric Disorders in General Practice.
Rutter, M., Tizzard, J. and Whitmore, K. (1970). "Education,
Health and Behaviour". Longman.
Shepherd, M., Cooper, B., Brown, A.C. and Kalton, G.W. (1966).
"Psychiatric Illness in General Practice". Oxford Medical
Publications.
Taylor Lord, S. and Chave, S. (1964). "Mental Health and
Environment". Long, London.
Wing, J.K. (1971). *British Journal of Hospital Medicine* **v**, 53.

SESSION III
DISCUSSION

Dr Brendan KELLY (Merthyr Tydfill): I started in general practice in South Wales about 20 years ago after considerable psychiatric experience. I found I could deal with neurotic patients just as well, and perhaps better than, hospitals. I did not want to do in daytime practice my specialty so I did it after hours. I started with 2 patients, but as the years went by numbers increased as I became aware of the patients needing this kind of treatment. So gradually we built up a group meeting on a Monday night for $3\frac{1}{2}$ hours after surgery. This went on for about 10 years. About 2 years ago the social services, with help, set up a unit in Merthyr which is staffed by one psychologist, 5 nurses and 3 social workers and I work there as a general practitioner. Referrals are either directly by the patients themselves, by patients' relatives or by anybody who has influence over patients. We all work equally within it as a public team, nobody taking the lead, but each one referring to the one whom they think can do best for the patient concerned.

Professor John COOPER: That is exactly the sort of thing that we know has been happening. I did emphasize that there was nothing new or unusual in the scheme which I was describing except that it is the first attempt to try it on a fairly large scale in a reasonably coherent community and a hospital.

Dr Godfrey FOWLER (Oxford): I particularly welcome Professor Cooper's initiative because it is in a teaching hospital. It has very important implications for medical education, that medical students should see the opportunities for consultants and general practitioners to co-operate. But although he has taken great trouble to match up his psychiatrists with his general practitioners, it must to some extent inhibit access of general practice to other psychiatrists. The GPs will refer patients to the particular psychiatrist attending their practices.

Professor COOPER: The possible disadvantages to the general practitioner of a limitation of his closely guarded right of

referral is a well known problem. In practice neither the
patients, nor most general practitioners, mind very much as
long as they get a good service and their patients are dealt
with fairly promptly. There are difficulties in zoning as well
as inhibiting referral to anyone preferred. And the GPs must
not be too disappointed if the psychiatrists equal out the
workload and do not see a particular patient.

Dr Thomas PASTOR (London): You mentioned a register of referrals. What do you document?

Professor COOPER: The case register automatically records all
psychiatric contacts in the area, outpatients, day care, domiciliary visits. It lists the facts of each incident of contact, where the referral has come from, the name of the doctor
or practice, etc. It is a fairly complete record which can be
analysed into the category of practice, a group of doctors or
a doctor, or the category of patients being referred in the
various ways. If there is any large scale effect of the
scheme on the pattern of services, the quality could change
without very much change in the quantity. The statistical
side is of interest but it is not the prime motivation for
the scheme.

Professor GOLDBERG: Could I ask Dr Ashton whether community
physicians are so preoccupied with administration that they
are now blaming family doctors for not doing the job that they
were meant to do themselves, namely preventive health?

Dr ASHTON: I agree with the sentiments behind the question.
There is totally inadequate recruitment into community medicine
as we need about 80 community physicians a year and we are
producing about 20.

Mrs Andrea POUND (Tavistock Clinic): I have been working for
the past 2 years on a community research project in the Kings
Health District, which is Camberwell and Peckham. We investigate depressed mothers and the effect of their depression on
their pre-school children. All the interviewing and conversa-
tions and so on are done in people's homes. Housing is easily
the most important factor in the mental health of most young
families. But if the father is sitting in the corner depressed
and with no likelihood of being employed, then unemployment
is the most important factor. What we ought to research is
not how to identify the mental illness in the community but
how to identify the factors in the community which make for
mental health.

Dr Judy GREENWOOD (Edinburgh): I was a GP for 10 years and
have now been a community psychiatrist for 10 years. At this
Conference we are all preaching to the converted as we hold

similar views, such as to train GPs in counselling skills, to share primary care and to pay more attention to long-term intervention. But in the real world, in most inner city areas the level of general practice and of provision of psychiatric services is actually pathetically low. We must decide what we can do over the next 5 year period, rather than waiting until the new GPs enter the system, which will not affect the joint services for at least 10 years.

Simple changes in the psychiatric service would reap lasting benefits. For example, the self-poisoning system of an area is little used as a means to teaching how to counsel, but most people admitted to a general hospital with an overdose are not psychiatrically ill but need counselling. We should be teaching our medical students and our psychiatric trainees how to counsel by using the patients. Finally by sectorizing psychiatry we give psychiatrists an opportunity to know their area, and their community, and to pass on their skills to the GPs.

PSYCHIATRIC RESEARCH IN GENERAL PRACTICE -
PAST, PRESENT AND FUTURE

Michael Shepherd

*Institute of Psychiatry, De Crespigny Park,
Denmark Hill, London, SE5*

SUMMARY

A brief review of post-war developments indicates why research
into psychiatric morbidity in primary care has been so poorly
developed. The theoretical and practical importance of such
work has nonetheless now been demonstrated and the major lines
of future inquiry are outlined.

Participants in so forward-looking a conference will understandably view the present, represented by the papers and discussions, as a guide to the future. But the present, as Thomas
Carlyle was fond of pointing out, is no more than a thin film
between the past and the future. In this instance the past
furnishes both lessons and guidelines for the future, and is
of some interest in its own right.

For convenience, I would drop anchor a generation ago. In
1953 the British Medical Journal devoted a leading editorial
to the theme of general practice research which was described
as being "in the air" (British Medical Journal, 1953). The
editorial reflected an opinion which had been summarized a
little earlier in a report of a College of General Practitioners Steering Committee:

> It is clear that there is a reawakening of interest in
> research work by doctors in general practice and in the
> possibilities of applying modern principles of scien-
> tific investigation to the problems of general practi-
> tioners (British Medical Journal, 1952).

I would underline the prefix in the word "reawakening".
Just over 100 years ago it was possible for the creator of
the finest portrait of a general practitioner in English literature to write:

> With our present rules and education, one must be satis-
> fied now and then to meet with a fair practitioner. As
> to the higher questions which determine the starting-
> point of a diagnosis - as to the philosophy of medical
> evidence - any glimmering of these can only come from
> a scientific culture of which country practitioners have
> no more notion than the man in the moon.

As always, George Eliot was painting an accurate picture of a
social situation, barely influenced by the past achievements
of outstanding individuals like Budd, Jenner and Withering.
Yet that same year of her comment, 1878, witnessed the confer-
ring of a degree on James Mackenzie who within a generation
was to demonstrate how the foundations of a clinical science
would be laid in a North country practice. Mackenzie's
achievement helped establish a model which was embodied in the
remarkably forward-looking Institute for Clinical Research
which he founded in 1919, one of its principal objectives
being the encouragement of general practitioners to participate
in scientific investigation. Like all truly original thinkers,
however, Mackenzie was far ahead of his time, and the implications of his work were to come into their own only in the post-
war years, when they could be buttressed by 2 major developments: the introduction of the National Health Service and
the creation of the College of General Practitioners.

The catalyst for the British Medical Journal editorial,
however, had been a recently published paper by the late Lord
Platt, entitled "Opportunities for research in general practice" (Platt, 1953), in which he made 2 points. The first of
these was that many investigations at the primary care level
are closely dependent on the use of medical statistics. A
lead in this direction had already been provided by Sir Austin
Bradford Hill in the course of his inquiries on behalf of the
British Medical Association into the services given by insurance
practitioners under the National Health Insurance Act and into
doctors' earnings (Hill, 1951). Large-scale studies of the
GPs' clinical activities had begun to appear, mostly from
workers with a public health orientation (Pemberton, 1949), and
it was in 1953 that the Chief Medical Statistician of the
General Register Office published the first of its studies on
general practitioners' records (General Register Office, 1953),
the precursor of the first National Morbidity Survey 5 years
later (General Register Office, 1958).

Platt's principal plea, however, was for practitioners
themselves to make use of the research potential at their dis-
posal and he illustrated his argument with a characteristically
pungent example:

The conventional picture of the research worker is that
of a rather austere man in a white coat with a background of complicated glassware. My idea of a research
worker, on the other hand, is a man who brushes his
teeth on the left side of his mouth only so as to use
the other side as a control and see if tooth-brushing
has any effect on the incidence of caries ... If he has
been badly educated in elementary principles he might
clean only his top teeth and not the bottom ones; but
that would admit a possible error of selection, for the
top and bottom sets, being morphologically different,
may differ inherently in their resistance to disease.
If he is a really good worker, on the other hand, he
will urge his brother - preferably an identical twin -
to clean only the right side and compare results.

The cultivation of this approach, as Platt went on to emphasize, becomes crucial because the spectrum of illnesses presented to the general practitioner is quite different from
that encountered in hospital and constitutes a special area of
inquiry in its own right. And prominent among these conditions
are the mental disorders which Sir James Mackintosh singled
out for particular attention in his own comments on research
in general practice at about the same time, a point picked up
by another lead-editorial on the subject, this time in the
Lancet:

The observation of years in a mental hospital or a psychiatric clinic may not reveal as much about such
patients in their true environment as the general practitioner learns in the course of his daily plodding
(Lancet, 1955).

Here, then, a generation ago was a challenge to the specialists
in mental disorders, and an opportunity for collaborative
research with the general practitioner. And yet, when I and
my colleagues initiated our own studies shortly afterwards we
were virtually alone in so doing.

Why should this have been the case? One clue can be derived
from the inaugural conference in 1952 of the Mental Health
Research Fund, as it was then called, which reflected contemporary opinion among senior investigators concerned with psychiatric research (Mental Health Research Fund, 1952). Their
stated objectives were, according to Sir Geoffrey Vickers, the
answers to 2 questions:

What are the ignorances which today principally hamper
our understanding of the nature, prevention, and care
of mental illness? What advances in research are most
likely to remove these, and so help to reduce the

population of mental hospitals and institutions for the
delinquents?

There was here an implicit assumption that mental disorder is
primarily the concern of the specialized mental health services,
and only Professor Tanner, in an aside, drew attention to the
fact that general practitioners had "access to material out of
reach to anyone else". That this material might contain a
segment of psychiatric morbidity which merited independent
investigation was evidently not deemed a topic for inquiry by
almost all members of the psychiatric establishment. That the
bulk of emotional disorders might fall outside the province
of the psychiatrist was simply not contemplated.

I would emphasize, however, that this negative or nescient
approach represented no more than a maintenance of pre-war
attitudes concerning the role of general practice in the
identification and management of mental disorder. As late as
1938, for example, the British Medical Association appointed
a Committee on Mental Health whose terms of references were:

> to inquire into and report upon the present medical
> equipment and provision for dealing with mental health
> in this country, with particular reference to the prob-
> lems of the treatment and prophylaxis of the psycho-
> neurotic and allied disorders (British Medical Associa-
> tion, 1941).

In the whole 40-page report there is virtually no mention of
primary care, apart from a single paragraph in the section on
incidence of mental disorder where the tone is as revealing
as the content:

> An attempt was made to obtain records of the incidence
> of psychoneurosis from a number of general practitioners
> who had at some time attended courses of lectures on
> the psychoneuroses for general practitioners, and who
> might therefore be expected to be interested in the sub-
> ject and to be competent to furnish useful information.
> Less than a dozen practitioners, however, were able to
> produce records, and the small number of patients seen
> and the variation in types of practice render the
> results of the inquiry statistically useless.

Not surprisingly, the Committee's "model scheme" for the
treatment of mental disorder failed to find any place at all
for the general practitioner.

Though the outbreak of World War II stimulated more interest
among psychiatrists in the mental health of the population at
large, it resulted in very little more appreciation of the
potential contribution of the family doctor. In 1942 a survey

was conducted by C.P. Blacker which carries particular significance because it was sponsored by the Ministry of Health,
whose Chief Medical Officer in his foreward to the consequent
publication referred pointedly to its potential value for
"the integration of the country's health services after the
war" (Jameson, 1946). These plans, however, barely involved
general practitioners who were even accused to being inade-
quately aware of and often prejudiced against the medical
health services.

   The same undercurrent is readily depicted in a brochure on
mental illness for general practitioners which was put together
by 7 senior psychiatrists for the Section of Social Psychiatry
of the Royal Medico-Psychological Association in 1946 (RMPA,
1946). Fortunately, perhaps, wiser counsels prevailed and
the material was never published. It turned out to be little
more than a clinical primer, written *de haut en bas*, which
a contemporary medical student would surely disdain. The
flavour may be derived from a sample contribution concerning
advice on those cases which might be appropriately referred
by the GP to the consultant psychiatrist:

   it is a sound rule to refer for diagnosis any patient
   who seeks advice for purely psychological symptoms such
   as fears, depression, convulsions - unless the doctor
   is able to spend sufficient time for a diagnostic interview himself.

It was true then and has remained true since that social and
community psychiatry, for which this country is probably best
known among mental health professionals, has been concerned
principally with the fate of either hospital in-patients who
are discharged into the community or with the extra-mural forms
of care. The standpoint has been summarized by one of its
foremost representatives who, after estimating that a population of 60,000 patients would yield 1,000 psychiatric patients
in the care of 3 psychiatrists, comments:

   There will also be about 24 family doctors in the area.
   These doctors, however, cannot give psychiatrists much
   help, for in our health service family doctors are
   already seeing the bulk of the patients with socio-
   economic problems (Bennett, 1973).

Against this background it is hardly surprising that while
recognizing emotional illness to be an important aspect of
primary care the Royal College of General Practitioners in
its early days should have turned to an alternative brand of
help offered in the form of the seminars organized by Michael
and Enid Balint from 1951 onwards at the Tavistock Clinic.
Drs Horder and Swift have documented the story of how this

teaching came to be incorporated in the College programme of vocational training and they go on to explain the reasons for its adoption:

> These seminars urged the continuing importance of the general practitioner's role at a time when specialization in clinical medicine looked like excluding it from the scene, and when the self-confidence of doctors doing this work was at its lowest. Concentrating on the patient's reaction to his disease, the contribution of feelings and interpersonal relationships to the production of symptoms, the patient's behaviour towards the doctor, and the doctor's feelings about the patient, they emphasized the "whole" patient at a time when every other powerful influence in medicine was fragmenting the patient into organ systems (or smaller parts). They thus reinstated a concern for the psychological and social aspects of medicine at a time when it was suspect and unfashionable, and helped to restore a balance which is today regarded as crucial to diagnosis and management in good general practice ... although these seminars may appear to have been an essay in psychiatric training of a limited type, based on psychoanalytic ideas, they did in fact reintroduce principles fundamental to the training of all doctors (Horder and Swift, 1979).

In one sense it may be contended that this comment constitutes an indictment of the neglect of general practice by the official representatives of psychological medicine. Matters have, of course, improved since then and joint committees between the 2 Royal Colleges have acknowledged common areas of interest in the spheres of education and manpower. Nonetheless, as Donald Hicks has pointed out in the splendid review of primary health care which he prepared for the DHSS (Hicks, 1976), it is apparent that whatever the role of the psychodynamic approach may have been in sustaining the self-confidence of general practitioners, its ideological infrastructure has not been conducive to the development of scientific research in the sphere of mental health. The same conclusion has been reached by other observers elsewhere and more recently the view of the general practitioner as a type of psychotherapist *manqué* has been challenged by practitioners themselves, most notably by Dr Peter Sowerby who, without underestimating the historical significance of the Balint seminars, cogently puts the case for a wider perspective:

> ... Michael Balint came to a false conclusion about the nature of a general practitioner's task, about the way

the problems posed by his difficult patients may be
identified, and about some of the training doctors
should receive. Balint's main contribution remains.
He showed us that scientific skills alone are not
enough if we are to understand our patients fully.
He also showed us how a descriptive science of human
behaviour in the consulting room was possible.
   To these insights must be added new understanding.
Popper has provided us with a clear line of demarca-
tion between science and the rest of our knowledge.
This idea suggests that general practitioners should
reaffirm the importance to them of the intellectual
discipline of science (Sowerby, 1977).

With this assertion Sowerby is going beyond the confines of
the debate over the claims made for and against a particular
point of view. He is taking a stand on the place of scientific
inquiry, and hence research, and facing up to a more fundamental issue implicit in the series of questions posed by T.H.
Pear 25 years ago:

   ... how far can the general practitioner be rigidly
   scientific ... and if he could and did, would he not
   become the "medical technician" of whom some doctors
   disapprove? Who would then deal with the patients'
   disabilities, inabilities, disorders, as distinct from
   narrowly defined "diseases"? And would the patient,
   qua patient, be allowed to be neurotic, or ever normally
   worried or subject to conflicts? Would the average
   doctor be happy if his "non-scientific" problems were
   handed over entirely to almoners, social workers,
   psychiatric social workers, marriage guidance counsellors, family welfare advisers, poor man's lawyers
   and specially selected priests? Most of these perform
   their functions excellently when properly chosen and
   trained, but would the increase in their responsibilities and numbers decrease those of the doctors, as
   we understand the term? (Pear, 1955).

Inasmuch as questions can be inverted statements Pear is
drawing attention here to the widely held but wholly false
notion that the caring doctor cannot be scientifically-minded,
a view which recalls the larger-scale debate on the assumptions
of clinical research in this country 50 years ago. Nowhere do
the issues arise more sharply than in the field of mental
ill-health at the primary care level, and they may be illustrated by another set of questions taken from a very different
context with an altogether different purpose, namely the mem-
bership examination of the Royal College of General

Practitioners. Here is a potted summary of the modified essay
question set in October 1980.

The case was that of Mr and Mrs Jones, an elderly married
couple aged 81 and 75 years respectively. After a lifetime
of good health Mrs Jones, the candidate is told, suffers a
transient cerebral episode from which she recovers completely.
She is found to be asymptomatic, but with a blood pressure of
210/125, and questions are asked, reasonably enough, about
diagnosis and treatment. Shortly afterwards Mr Jones develops
a persistent low backache which calls for assessment. At the
same time Mrs Jones is described as "clearly unhappy", "at
the end of her tether", "unable to cope" and the candidate is
asked to suggest why this should be so and what he should do.
Mr Jones is found to be suffering from Paget's disease with
some rather curious laboratory findings which prompt further
questioning. Shortly afterwards he is said to be apathetic,
confused and without the will to live, while his wife appears
to be "extremely agitated". Next day he is found wandering
at 2 a.m. in the snow dressed in his pyjamas; he contracts
bronchopneumonia, is admitted to hospital and dies. The questions to the candidate, however, then concern the widow, as
follows:

> You visit Mrs Jones at home a few days later. Her son
> and daughter-in-law are with her. She is smiling and
> talking animatedly but she recognizes and welcomes you.
> You are given a cup of tea and left alone with her. You
> decide to direct the conversation to her feelings about
> her husband's death and her own future. What are the
> advantages and disadvantages of this approach? What
> problems might you anticipate with Mrs Jones in the next
> year or two?

A case-history of this type illustrates an awareness of the
need to take account of the social setting of psychiatric
morbidity in general practice, the inter-relationships of
physical and psychological ill-health and the assessment of
psychiatric morbidity under stress. But while the questions
on, say, Mr Jones' Paget's disease and his bronchopneumonia
can be answered by reference to a large, established store of
knowledge, the answers to the problems posed by Mrs Jones are
much less well-established. The candidate will find conflict-
ing opinions in the text books on the nature of her mental
state, the justification for discussing her feelings and her
ultimate prognosis.

Such questions belong a large range of problems which call
for the intensive study of mental disorder in a primary care
setting. In the light of what we can now recognize as a
large and potentially vital area of inquiry the work conducted

so far must, in my view, be accounted sadly inadequate, even
if there are good historical reasons for the deficiency. The
methods required are both epidemiological and clinical, and
some of the studies presented at this meeting provide a cross-
section of work in progress which holds out encouraging prospects for future research. These inquiries will impinge on
some of the major topics in psychological medicine. Among
these I would mention, first, the pressing need to examine the
whole concept of neurosis, a term which has already been dropped
from the latest version of the American Diagnostic and Statistical Manual as out-moded and operationally sterile (American
Psychiatric Association, 1980), and calls for re-assessment of
its clinical, behavioural and social components. More information on the causal factors and outcome of "neurotic" illness,
and especially the minor affective disorders, is of particular
significance in view of their demonstrated prevalence. For
this purpose the general practitioner is well-placed to assume
the dual roles of clinical epidemiologist and clinical anthro-
polist in the investigation of several relevant issues, including the relationship of distress to depression, personality-
traits to personality-disorders, and also of particular symptom
patterns like eating behaviour to eating disorders and of
drinking-patterns to alcohol-related morbidity.

Here he would be doing no more than address himself to the
task so clearly defined by James Mackenzie:

To utilize the opportunities of a general practitioner
to study the earliest symptoms of disease, and the
bearings of the disease upon the patient's future life.

In pursuit of his inquiries, however, he will have to leave
the safe confines of his consulting room and enter the wilder-
ness of the community at large where he is likely to encounter
a small platoon of psychiatric epidemiologists who are currently
on safari, armed with questionnaires and computer programmes,
in search of the unicorn of "caseness", regardless of the
warning from one of their fellow-travellers that "the concept
of a "case" is a chimaera existing only in the mind of the
observer" (Copeland, 1981). One hopes that the 2 parties may
learn from each other, a prospect which will be improved if
they recall that psychiatric illness at this level of identification is so deeply embedded in social pathology as to
demand a medico-social approach *ab initio*, with profound
implications for classification.

Closely related to diagnosis and outcome is treatment, and
in particular the prospects for therapeutic evaluation. Here
a lead has been taken by the large-scale MRC trial of the
treatment of mild to moderate hypertension which involved the
collaboration of nearly 200 general practices over the whole

country. The chairman of the working party responsible for
the trial's co-ordination has spelt out its wider implications:

> The hardest part was discovering the right type of
> organization, which made it possible to build on the
> strength of general practice by providing the necessary
> extra supporting staff and funding. Since I consider
> this lesson is more important than the results of the
> trial itself, I hope that it will have considerable
> influence on the thinking of the DHSS and the MRC.
> General practice organization is well-suited for par-
> ticipation in drug assessments, and the speed and
> validity of the answers about actions and side-effects
> of drugs could be vastly improved. All parties would
> benefit (Peart, 1980).

I cannot, of course, speak for the thinking within either the
DHSS or the MRC but it is encouraging to know that the network
of general practitioners may shortly be engaged in a dominantly
psychiatric investigation. One may hope that a study of this
type will demonstrate the value of large-scale, multi-centred
investigations in the same way as the now classical MCR study
of the treatment of hospitalized depressive illness in the
mid-1960s (Medical Research Council, 1965). It may even render
feasible the examination of the role of the primary care
physician in the prevention of mental disorder, as claimed –
but hardly demonstrated – in the recently published document
of the Royal College of General Practitioners (Royal College
of General Practitioners, 1981).

The other broad field of future research which calls for
development is the organization of health services. The
national deployment of the resources of the NHS should clearly
be more closely linked to a knowledge of disease rather than
to the tides of administrative fashion but it is worth
recalling the conclusions of a WHO Group which surveyed the
field in several European countries some years ago to reach
the conclusion that:

> The crucial question is not how the general practitioner
> can fit into the mental health services but rather how
> the psychiatrist can collaborate most effectively with
> primary medical services and reinforce the effectiveness
> of the primary physician as a member of the mental
> health team (WHO, 1973).

Recently, there are signs that the same verdict has been
reached in North America despite its long-standing emphasis on
hospital medicine (Institute of Medicine, 1979), but a programme conceived *de bas en haut* will be needed if this aim is
to be realized.

At the same time it has to be underlined that the recognition of the importance of the psychosocial dimension of
morbidity in general practice and of its impact on the primary
care team does not necessarily lead to appropriate action, and
that the key attitudes involved are those of general practitioners as well as of psychiatrists. This issue has been
given substance by the results of the second study of general
practice carried out by Ann Cartwright and her colleagues at
the Institute for Social Studies in Medical Care (Cartwright
and Anderson, 1981). The information was derived from the
responses of 1,000 individuals related to those of their GPs.
Surprisingly, few differences were detected in the views of
either group of respondents when compared with those of 2
similar groups in 1964, but in 2 respects the situation had
clearly deteriorated. One of these concerns home-visiting,
with which we are not directly concerned; the other is best
summarized in Cartwright's own words:

> Both doctors and patients were less likely in 1977 than
> in 1964 to regard it as appropriate for patients to
> consult their general practitioner about problems in
> their family lives. At the same time many doctors felt
> there was a growing tendency for people to look to them
> for this sort of help ... The deterioration in the
> service indicated by doctors' unwillingness to accept
> the social content of their work and the lack of improve-
> ment in attitudes to "trivial" consultations are more
> surprising because it would seem from reading the
> Journal of the Royal College of General Practitioners
> and the writings of doctors in academic departments of
> general practice that more emphasis and attention is
> being placed on learning to care, and less on a mech-
> anistic model ... But doctors who are vocal in the
> press and universities are likely to be atypical and a
> picture of their attitudes will give a mistaken impres-
> sion of a renaissance in general practice ... The total
> picture may well be more gloomy than our study suggests.

The recent report on primary care in London bears out this
finding (London Health Planning Consortium, 1981) and the
precise role of other members of the primary care team remains
an important task for the future, even at a time when economic
stringencies have so affected the NHS that primary care
doctor has been seen as "picking up the pieces of the hospital
services" (Guardian, 1981).
     It is now evident that all these and many other related
questions are susceptible to research involving primary care
workers and mental health specialists. J.G. Howie, who
has analysed the nature of some 400 publications by GPs over

a 5-year period in the 1970s, sub-divides the categories of research into 5 groups:

therapeutic assessment of drugs and other modalities of treatment, natural history studies of individual illnesses, activities in the fields of prevention, screening or education, diagnostic and management decisions and practice organization (including team-care, record-keeping, workload, etc.) (Howie, 1979).

Of these studies a relatively small number have so far been devoted to psychiatric problems. The case for intensive investigation along a broad front has now been established, but it must be acknowledged that so far we have barely scratched the surface. If it serves any one purpose this conference will, I hope, initiate a concerted and large-scale research effort in a major but poorly developed field of inquiry.

REFERENCES

American Psychiatric Association (1980). Diagnostic and Statistical Manual of Mental Disorders (3rd edition), Washington, D.C.

Bennett, D.H. (1973). Community mental health services in Britain. *American Journal of Psychiatry* **130**, 1065-1070.

British Medical Association (1941). Report of Committee on Mental Health. B.M.A., London.

British Medical Journal (1952). Report of General Practice Steering Committee **2**, 1321.

British Medical Journal (1953). Research in general practice (editorial), **i**, 605-606.

Cartwright, A. and Anderson, R. (1981). "General Practice Revisited" . Tavistock Publications, London.

Copeland, J. (1981). What is a "case"? A case for what?. *In* "What is a Case?" (Eds J.K. Wing, P. Bebbington and L.N. Robins. p.9. Grant McIntyre, London.

General Register Office (1953). General Practitioners' Records. Studies on Medical and Population Subjects, No.7. HMSO, London.

General Register Office (1958). Morbidity Statistics from General Practice. Vol.1. Studies on Medical and Population Subjects, No.14. HMSO, London.

The Guardian (1981). Dr Procrustes prescribes. September 12, p.12.

Hicks, D. (1976). Primary Health Care. HMSO, London.

Hill, A.B. (1951). The doctor's day and pay. *Journal of the Royal Statistical Society*, Series A (General), **114**, 1.

Horder, J.P. and Swift, G. (1979). The history of vocational training for general practice. *Journal of the Royal College of General Practitioners* **29**, 24-32.

Howie, J.G.R. (1979). "Research in General Practice". Croom Helm, London.

Institute of Medicine, National Academy of Sciences (1979). Conference Report. Mental Health Services in General Health Care, Vol. I. Washington, D.C.

Jameson, W. (1946). Foreword. *In* "Neurosis and the Mental Health Services" (Ed. C.P. Blacker), p.v. Oxford University Press, London.

Lancet (1952). Medical Conferences: Projects for Research on Mental Health. **i**, 664-666.

Lancet (1955). Research in General Practice (editorial), **ii**, 953-954.

London Health Planning Consortium (1981). Primary Health Care in Inner London. Report of a Study Group. London.

Medical Research Council (1965). Report by its Clinical Committee: clinical trial of the treatment of depression. *British Medical Journal* **i**, 881-886.

Pear, T.H. (1955). "Social Differences in English Life". p.39. Allen and Unwin, London.

Peart, W.S. (1980). The pharmaceutical industry: research and responsibility. *Lancet* **ii**, 465-466.

Pemberton, J. (1949). Illness in general practice. *British Medical Journal* **i**, 306-308.

Platt, H.R. (1953). Opportunities for research in general practice. *British Medical Journal* **i**, 577-580.

Royal College of General Practitioners (1981). Report from General Practice 20. Prevention of Psychiatric Disorders in General Practice. London.

The Royal Medico-Psychological Association (1946). Brochure for General Practitioners (unpublished).

Shepherd, M., Cooper, B., Brown, A.C., Kalton, G.W. and Clare, A.W. (1981). "Psychiatric Illness in General Practice. 2nd edition". Oxford University Press, Oxford.

Sowerby, P. (1977). Balint reassessed. *Journal of the Royal College of General Practitioners* **27**, 583-589.

World Health Organization (1973). Report of Working Group. Psychiatry and Primary Medical Care. Copenhagen.

The CHAIRMAN: We have been told about the continuum basis
rather than the categorical basis of mental illness. But it
is more complicated than that because these continua interact.
For example, vulnerability has subordinate categories within
it such as the personal vulnerability of the psychologist and
the psychiatrist and the sociological vulnerability that
Brown and others discuss. Thus the picture is very complex,
both at the research level and at the clinical level, which
involves an element of pattern recognition. But the GP is
ideally situated for that pattern recognition because the facts
do not have to be elicited by questionnaire and history taking
and so on but are part of the life of the individual.
     Another important point is that normal emotional stress is
not necessarily less severe than the pathological. For example
the melancholy apathy of the adolescent when things go wrong
is quite severe depression but entirely normal. It is part
of the development of the individual from which develops the
coping mechanism. So it would be wrong to rob the adolescent
of these experiences by pharmacological intervention and one
must deal with them in a manner that allows these coping
mechanisms to develop.

Mrs Roslyn CORNEY (London): Cases of bereavement, who have
been sedated for some months after the event to get a good
night's sleep are much harder to deal with later.

Dr Anthony CLIFT (Manchester): Could Professor Shepherd tell
us the type of research ventures which would be appropriate
for a doctor working with his own patients and from which good
statistical results are feasible?

Dr John HALL (Oxford): Throughout the conference there has
been reference to the involvement of other professions with
general practitioners, including psychologists, social workers,
health visitors, counsellors, etc. This implies some skills
which GPs lack and which they perceive to be present in these
other professions. GPs may be looking for particular skills
from particular professions and actually be uncertain which

particular profession offers those skills. Careful analysis
of the supporting skills is needed to help GPs. There are
several examples of the role change in other health care
professions. Health educators were introduced several years
ago and have taken over some areas previously covered by health
visitors. Other examples are the community psychiatric nurse
and the nurse therapist. The Jay Report contained a serious
suggestion that one area of nursing should cease to be nursing
and become a branch of social work. There are 2 implications:
first, if we can analyse those skills it will affect the
training of a wide range of other professions; and second, we
may need a major regrouping of health care professionals to
meet general practitioners' needs.

Dr John HORDER: I want to raise the question of time. Is one
of the "skills" which other professions have and which we lack
really that they have more time. Our mean consultation time
is 6 or 7 minutes, the French have 13 and the Americans at
least 18. Patients complain that we do not listen to them,
the doctor has not got time. It is also worrying general
practitioners who feel that they do not have the time to do
the things they know how to do. This results from better
training because they know how to do more things and how to do
them better.

Dr Thomas PASTOR (London): Could Professor Shepherd tell us
what work has been done in looking at what exists amongst GPs
re the skills available to them?

The CHAIRMAN: Of course, there are economic and manpower
factors underlying this particular question.

Dr Andrew MARKUS (Thames): To take up Dr Horder's point, some
time ago when we felt pressed in our practice with a 3 in 20
minute appointment system, we actually extended it to a 10
minute appointment system. We actually reduced our consultation rate over the year, from an average of 2.75 per person
on the list per annum to 2.5, a drop of about 10%. However,
the actual time that we increased the consultation by was
about 30%. So we spend more time with our patients as a
result of this move than we did before. Hopefully, we have
given better care, but we do not know.

Dr June HUNTINGTON (Sydney, Australia): I know from informal
contact with a group practice in Sydney that they too have been
deliberately lengthening consultations. They see it as good
practice. Their early findings are that the consultation rate
of patients over the year falls when they are actually given
more time.
    A lot more research needs to be done on patients who bring

psychosocial problems, trying to link the type of problem they have to the type of skill needed to deal with it. My own experience of general practice suggests that not all general practitioners want to be a healer as one who listens or who reflects back to the person. Nor do all people who come into the surgery want a healer. My social worker seemed a better healer for the people who wanted a healer than did most of the doctors.

I would like to encourage the GPs here to think about general practice as a base for community work, whether it is they who do it or whether it is health visitors or social workers who do it. I was quite amazed in my own project in Sydney at the way in which the social worker was able to identify patients with complementary needs. For example, somebody had lost their Scrabble partner through death. Another patient said to the social worker that she would like somebody to play Scrabble with and the 2 met up.

Dr John REA (Kentish Town, London): Ann Cartwright wrote in 1977 that more doctors were feeling frustrated that they lacked enough time for their consultations than had been the case 13 years before. She also pointed out that where there was an attached social worker the doctors did not perceive fewer of their patients as having trivial or inappropriate problems, but rather the reverse. The reason they were feeling more frustrated was because the problems presented to them were outside their training.

Dr WHITFIELD (Bristol): I would like to sound a word of warning, based on our own experience in Bristol. Two years ago we circularized all general practitioners with a questionnaire based on Professor Shepherd's questionnaire, and asked them, inter alia, "Would you like a consultant psychiatrist to visit you in your surgery on a regular basis and discuss patients with you?" Only 33% of the general practitioners who replied said they would; 44% said "No". Thus, a large number of general practitioners do not seek co-operation with psychiatrists.

Dr John PRICE (Birmingham): What matters is my faith in the people I work with, how I trust them and how I get on with them. Our local mental hospital is changing its policies and discharging many patients. Stress developed in those working with them and we had to help lessen the stress in those caring workers by setting up a small group of a psychiatrist, a social worker, a hospital chaplain with marriage guidance experience and a GP. The patient or family or the worker came along and was able to obtain help and backing. This started preventive psychiatry for the workers themselves!

Dr Ian BERG (Leeds): Would Professor Shepherd comment on the
role of technology in psychiatry in general practice, because
it seems to me increasingly machines are being used to collect
information.

Dr Alexis BROOK (London): John Horder showed that a few
patients caused a disproportionately large workload in general
practice. Is this not a particular area that requires
research attention by a combined approach from GPs and psychiatrists to look at that particular group? Some of the patients
in the group referred to by June Huntington are people of that
type who go because they get some relief by using their doctor
as a receptacle to offload their worries, leaving him feeling
worried and confused and uncertain how to cope while they go
out feeling a bit better.

Professor SHEPHERD: Only a few questions were directed at me
personally. First, what should a GP actually do if he wants
to carry out research. Nowadays, particularly if he is working
in a group practice, the number of questions is almost infinite.
For example, in the psychiatric field, John Fry has been
publishing for 25 years studies based entirely on his own
practice. We have been very closely involved with him as we
are not entirely epidemiological in our orientation and we do
work with individual doctors. But these studies depend on the
ability of individual doctors to keep records, and to keep
those as John Fry does, is something which in my experience
is very rare. The question of time which John Horder raises
can be overcome by using the facilities and goodwill of whatever university department is available. A good example is the
study which we have recently done with John Fry. All his
patients who are diagnosed by him as having some form of
psychiatric disorder 20 years ago were followed up. There is
no other way one could get a carefully monitored natural
history study over a biological span of 20 years with patients
like this. All he needed was advice on computerization and
a bit of help with the organization of the data, but the data
were collected by him.

   The last question was concerning computers. One of my
colleagues has been using computerized methods for psychiatric
diagnosis and is presently preparing to see whether they can
be introduced into the primary care situation. It is, of
course, fraught with difficulties but it was inevitable that
when the technology came along somebody was going to try to
use it.

SUBJECT INDEX